Guidelines for trauma quality improvement programmes

WORLD HEALTH ORGANIZATION

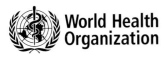

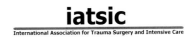

INTERNATIONAL SOCIETY OF SURGERY
SOCIÉTÉ INTERNATIONALE DE CHIRURGIE
and
INTERNATIONAL ASSOCIATION FOR TRAUMA SURGERY
AND INTENSIVE CARE

WHO Library Cataloguing-in-Publication Data

1.Wounds and injuries - therapy. 2.Wounds and injuries - prevention and control. 3.Delivery of health care - organization and administration. 4.Emergency medical services - organization and administration. 5.Emergency medical services - standards. I.World Health Organization. Dept. of Violence and Injury Prevention and Disability. II.International Association for Trauma Surgery and Intensive Care. III.International Society of Surgery.

ISBN 978 92 4 159774 6   (NLM classification: WO 700)

Printed in Malta

Contents

Preface

Injury is a major public health problem. Each year, 5.8 million people die from injury, and many more are disabled. The burden is especially high in low-income and middle-income countries, where over 90% of injury deaths occur. To lower this unacceptable burden, a spectrum of actions is needed, including better surveillance and research, increased implementation of road safety and other forms of injury prevention, and strengthening of the current scenario in trauma care (care of the injured). Many high-income countries have significantly lowered trauma mortality rates by improving the organization of, and planning for, trauma care through implementation of trauma systems that address all aspects of care – from the prehospital setting, to initial resuscitation in the hospital, to longer term definitive care. Such organized trauma systems have been only minimally implemented in most low-income and middle-income countries.

In order to promote greater implementation of effective, affordable, and sustainable trauma systems globally, the World Health Organization (WHO) and the International Association for Trauma Surgery and Intensive Care (IATSIC) have worked collaboratively in the past to produce *Guidelines for essential trauma care*, which defined the core essential trauma care services that every injured person in the world should realistically be able to receive, even in the lowest income setting. In order to assure the availability of these services, that publication went on to propose the minimum human resources, physical resources, and administrative mechanisms that should be in place in the range of health care facilities globally. That publication and the related *Prehospital trauma care systems* have considerably catalysed improvements in trauma systems in many countries since their release several years ago.

Efforts to strengthen trauma care globally have also received a considerable boost from the adoption of World Health Assembly Resolution WHA60.22 on trauma and emergency care services which called on governments and WHO to increase their efforts to strengthen services for victims of trauma and other medical emergencies. Among other provisions, this resolution specifically called upon WHO "to provide support to Member States for design of quality-improvement programmes" on trauma care. Quality improvement programmes have been an integral part of trauma systems in high-income countries and have shown considerable promise in the small number of locations in low-income and middle-income countries in which they have been utilized.

In order to contribute to implementation of the World Health Assembly resolution, WHO and IATSIC have expanded their collaborative work to produce this guideline on trauma quality improvement. This document seeks to provide how-to-do guidance to support efforts to establish quality improvement programmes for trauma care. It covers a range of techniques, but it emphasizes basic methods that are applicable to all countries globally. These guidelines have been developed collaboratively by our two organizations, along with input from many experts who are actively involved in the care of injured persons worldwide, including several pioneers in the adaptation of quality improvement methods to the realities of low-income and middle-income countries.

In addition to providing technical guidance, these guidelines are intended to stimulate the growth of quality improvement programmes globally and to stimulate greater collaboration between those involved in these programmes and those involved with synergistic efforts to promote greater patient safety and to strengthen health care systems overall. We encourage all who are involved in providing, administering, or planning trauma care services to implement the recommendations contained in these guidelines.

Etienne Krug, MD, MPH
Director,
Department of Violence and Injury
Prevention and Disability,
WHO, Geneva

Ian Civil, MBChB, FRACS, FACS
Director,
Auckland City Hospital Trauma
Services
Auckland, New Zealand
President, IATSIC

Contributors

Editors

Charles Mock, Catherine Juillard, Susan Brundage, Jacques Goosen, Manjul Joshipura

Critical readers of the guidelines (excluding editors)

Maia Ambegaokar, Raed Arafat, Carlos Arreola Risa, Kenneth Boffard, Gerard Castro, Witaya Chadbunchachai, Ian Civil, Gerald Dziekan, Dominique Egger, Ranjith Ellawala, Thomas Esposito, Atul Gawande, Russell Gruen, Laura Hawken, Vikas Kapil, Christine Keyes, Etienne Krug, Ari Leppaniemi, Ronald Maier, Marcos Musafir, Thai Son Nguyen, Eric Ossmann, Andres Rubiano, Potipong Ruengjui, Scott Sasser, Sandro Scarpelini, Heather Sherman, Mathew Varghese, Ahmed Zakariah

Additional contributors to boxes and tables

Witaya Chanbunchachai (Box 1), Russell Gruen (Table 16), Ronald Maier (Table 15)

None of the experts involved in the development of this publication declared any conflict of interest.

Acknowledgements

The World Health Organization, the International Association for Trauma Surgery and Intensive Care, and the editorial committee acknowledge with thanks the reviewers and contributors whose dedication, support and expertise made these guidelines possible.

The guidelines also benefited from the contributions of a number of other people. In particular, acknowledgement is made to Avery Nathens and Melanie Neal for advice on risk adjustment methods; David Bramley for editorial assistance; Irene Lengui for design of the cover and layout; and Pascale Lanvers, Claire Scheurer, and Hélène Dufays for administrative support.

The World Health Organization and the editorial committee also wish to thank the following for providing funding for the development, writing and publication of this document: the United States Centers for Disease Control and Prevention, the World Bank, and the International Association for Trauma Surgery and Intensive Care.

Executive Summary

The response to the growing problem of injury needs to include the improvement of care of the injured (i.e. trauma care). Quality improvement (QI) programmes offer an affordable and sustainable means to implement such improvements. These programmes enable health care institutions to better monitor trauma care services, better detect problems in care, and more effectively enact and evaluate corrective measures targeted at these problems. In so doing, many deaths of injury victims can be avoided.

The goal of this publication is to give guidance on ways in which health care institutions globally can implement QI programmes oriented to strengthening care of the injured. This guidance is intended to be universally applicable to all countries, no matter what their economic level.

These guidelines provide basic definitions and an overview of the field of QI, so that those not familiar with this field will have a working knowledge of it. Evidence of the benefit of QI in general and trauma QI in particular is then laid out. The main part of the publication reviews the most common methods of trauma QI, written in a how-to-do fashion. This covers a wide range of techniques. The first two of these are especially emphasized as ways in which to strengthen trauma QI in the setting of low-income and middle-income countries.

First are morbidity and mortality (M & M) conferences. These are already being regularly conducted in many hospitals worldwide, but often they are not well utilized to achieve the goal of improving trauma care. Several improvements could change this. These include more attention to detail in the procedures for conducting the conference, such as scheduling, optimizing the length of the M & M meeting, defining who should attend and who should run the meeting, as well as assuring the types of cases that should be reviewed. Needed improvements also include more attention to detail in identifying problems (especially those relating to systems issues), developing reasonable corrective action plans, following through on implementing these plans, and evaluating whether the corrective action has had its intended consequences. Several structural issues could also increase the effectiveness of M & M conferences. These include availability of adequate support staff for logistics and data management, as well assuring active participation and buy-in by a wide range of clinicians involved with trauma care.

Second are preventable death panel reviews. These provide for more formal input as to determination of preventability of trauma deaths and identification of factors of care that need to be strengthened. Such input is obtained from a range of clinicians whose involvement not only provides multidisciplinary technical expertise but also investment in the successful conduct of corrective actions that are identified. These guidelines provide how-to-do guidance on constituting the panel, preparing data for the review, conducting the case review process, and documenting and analysing the case discussions. Both M & M conferences and preventable death panel reviews are eminently feasible and widely applicable, and are especially of relevance to strengthening of care of the injured in low-income and middle-income countries.

More advanced QI techniques are also covered. One of these is the use of the medical records system to monitor specific variables, known as audit filters. These provide objective data on the occurrence and rates of potential problems, which can then be monitored as corrective measures are put in place. These audit filters can include process-of-care measures, as well as complications, errors, adverse events, and sentinel events.

Other more advanced QI methods include statistical techniques for severity adjustment. These include use of a number of different anatomical and physiological injury scoring systems that help to compare injuries between patients objectively. These scoring methods assist QI programmes by allowing them to focus on patients who die with low injury severity (e.g. medically preventable deaths) and by allowing programmes to compare the outcome of large groups of patients against established norms.

Common to all the above techniques is that they should lead to implementation of corrective strategies to fix problems that are identified, they should monitor the effectiveness of such corrective strategies, and they should assure that these corrective strategies have had their intended effect (i.e. closing the loop). Several types of corrective strategies can be utilized, including: guidelines, pathways, and protocols; targeted education; actions targeted at specific providers; and enhanced resources, facilities, or communication.

The techniques discussed are applicable to a wide range of circumstances. However, special issues arise in using QI to address system-wide and prehospital trauma care. These include specific measures of quality that need to be monitored, specific types of monitoring methods, and specific corrective actions.

All of the techniques of QI rely on adequate data. In many circumstances there is a need to address improvements in data collection and usage to better assure timely, reliable, and adequate data on which to base QI activities. This may imply better recording of data at the time of patient presentation. It may imply better handling and availability of that data from standard medical record systems. In some circumstances, it may imply the establishment of a formal trauma registry, which can be done in an affordable, sustainable and simple fashion.

These guidelines end with discussion of the appropriateness of different techniques at different levels of the health care system, and of the overlap with other related activities such as clinical algorithms for trauma care, efforts to promote patient safety, and efforts to strengthen health care management. Finally, in the annexes, several case examples are provided for practice in scrutinizing clinical data, identifying problems in care, and deriving practical and effective corrective strategies.

In summary, this document provides how-to-do guidance on a range of different trauma QI methods. These are broadly applicable to all health care institutions that care for the injured in countries at all economic levels. One or more of the methods described in this document will be directly applicable to any given institution and will enable that institution to upgrade the level of function of its existing trauma QI activities. In so doing, the quality of trauma care can be strengthened and the lives of many injured persons saved.

1. Introduction

Injury[1] is a leading cause of death and disability worldwide. Responses to this problem must encompass both prevention and improvements in the care of injury victims. Much needs to be done globally to strengthen care of the injured. This can be accomplished in an affordable and sustainable manner especially by improving the organization of, and planning for, trauma care services. Quality improvement (QI) programmes offer a means to accomplish such improved organization and planning. These programmes provide hard data on both what is working well and what is not working well and needs to be improved.

Unfortunately, trauma QI programmes are insufficiently utilized globally. The World Health Assembly recently called for greater usage of such programmes. In Resolution WHA60.22 on trauma and emergency care services, the World Health Assembly specifically called on WHO to "to provide support to Member States for design of quality-improvement programmes" on trauma care. This publication is a result of that request.

This publication seeks to give guidance on ways in which health care institutions globally can strengthen the trauma care they provide through implementation of QI programmes. This guidance is intended to be universally applicable to all countries, no matter what their economic level, but is especially oriented to the circumstances of low-income and middle-income countries. Moreover, this publication is also intended to provide a stimulus for more widespread adoption of trauma QI programmes globally.

The recommendations contained in these guidelines have been drawn up through collaboration between:

- the Department of Violence and Injury Prevention and Disability (VIP) at WHO;
- the International Association for Trauma Surgery and Intensive Care

---

[1] The terms "injury" and "trauma" are used interchangeably throughout these guidelines.

4

(IATSIC), which is an integrated society within the broader International Society of Surgery/Société Internationale de Chirurgie (ISS/SIC);
- members of WHO's Trauma and Emergency Care Services (TECS) advisory group, which includes people active in providing or administering trauma care services in countries around the world, including many from Africa, Asia, and Latin America.

The target audience for these guidelines include planners in ministries of health, hospital administrators, nursing service directors, medical service directors and clinicians, both individually and collectively, through organizations such as societies of surgery, anaesthesia, traumatology and other disciplines that deal with the injured patient. These guidelines are relevant to both those working in prehospital trauma care and those involved with care at fixed facilities. Likewise, they are relevant to those working in countries at all economic levels. Broadly construed, the guidelines are of relevance to anyone involved in providing or administering trauma care services. They can be put to use by such persons as a means to better accomplish their work of strengthening care of the injured, through the improved organization and planning that QI programmes offer. It is anticipated that these guidelines will remain relevant for at least 10 years after publication.

2. Overview of quality improvement

This publication starts with definitions and with an overview of QI and its basic elements, so that those not familiar with this field may obtain a working knowledge of it.

2.1 Definitions and basics of quality improvement

Quality of care is characterized as "the degree to which health services for individuals and populations increase the likelihood of desired health outcomes and are consistent with the current professional knowledge" (Institute of Medicine, 1999). QI can be defined as the optimization of resources – including knowledge, practical skills and material assets to produce good health. QI is a method of improving medical care by monitoring the elements of diagnosis, treatment and outcome. QI involves both prospective and retrospective review and is aimed at advancement towards improved outcomes – measuring the current status and figuring out ways to make care better. QI evaluates the performance of both individual providers and the systems in which they work (Institute of Medicine, 2001a; Institute of Medicine, 2001b; Maier and Rhodes, 2001; Ko, Maggard and Agustin, 2005; Peabody et al., 2006).

Assessment and monitoring of quality in health care has evolved considerably over the past 100 years and has been given many different names and their associated acronyms (Table 1). During this time, there has been a shift in the mindset with which the medical community has approached the topic. One of the original strategies introduced to improve the quality of medical care, termed the "medical audit", originated in the 19th and early 20th centuries and consisted of a system for counting procedures, complications and deaths. This approach was similar to the subsequent "quality assurance" (QA). These earlier approaches were directed primarily towards defining standards of performance in medical care and identifying unacceptable levels of doctor performance in achieving these standards.

These earlier approaches often involved determining fault after something went wrong. From this context, QA was viewed as reactive, policing, apportioning

TABLE 1 **The evolution of terminology for quality improvement**

Timeline	Term	Definition
1900s	Medical Audit (MA)	A detailed *review* and *evaluation* of selected *clinical records* by qualified professional personnel for evaluating quality of *medical care*.
1920s	Quality Assurance (QA)	A planned and systematic set of activities undertaken to ensure that standards and procedures are adhered to and that delivered products or services meet performance requirements.
1980s	Total Quality Management (TQM)	An organizational management approach that consists of making all individuals responsible for improving the quality of health care. The TQM approach to quality assurance emphasizes continuous product or service improvements through involvement of the workforce.
	Continuous Quality Improvement (CQI)	A management approach to improving and maintaining quality that emphasizes internally driven and relatively continuous assessments of potential causes of quality defects, followed by action aimed either at avoiding decrease in quality or at correcting it at an early stage.
1990s	Performance Improvement (PI)	"The continuous evaluation of a system and the providers through structured review of the process of care as well as outcomes" (Maier and Rhodes, 2001). PI has evolved from previous quality assurance paradigms and represents a more scientific and evidence-based continuation of those standards.
2000s	Quality Improvement (QI)	A method of evaluating and improving processes of patient care which emphasizes a multidisciplinary approach to problem-solving, and which focuses not on individuals but on systems of patient care that may be the cause of variations. QI consists of periodic scheduled evaluation of organizational activities, policies, procedures and performance to identify best practices and target areas in need of improvement and includes implementation of corrective actions or policy changes where needed.

References: Institute of Medicine, 2001b; Maier and Rhodes, 2001; American College of Surgeons, 2006

blame, and even punitive. The medical community developed negative perceptions of these activities and often resisted their implementation.

Thus, it has been necessary to shift the focus away from the individual providers and their errors to a system-wide perspective. A pioneer who worked to accomplish this was Avedis Donabedian. He prompted a shift from focusing on the assessment of QA that centered on "doctor or human" performance to a more sophisticated model that embraced two major fundamental concepts – "systems" measures and "human" measures – in order to achieve optimal patient outcomes. This novel approach destigmatized the individual as a target to "blame" for unfavourable outcomes and emphasized a broader understanding in that QA requires awareness that the system also contributes to error. The model defined by Donabedian involves three concepts – structure, process, and outcomes (Donabedian, 1996) (Table 2).

TABLE 2 **Three elements of quality**

Quality comprises three elements:
Structure refers to stable, material characteristics (infrastructure, tools, technology) and the resources of the organizations that provide care and the financing of care (levels of funding, staffing, training, skills, payment schemes, incentives).
Process is the interaction between care-givers and patients during which structural inputs from the health care system are transformed into health outcomes. The process is the actual provision of medical care to the patient.
Outcomes can be measured in terms of health status, deaths, or disability-adjusted life years – a measure that encompasses the morbidity and mortality of patients or groups of patients. Outcomes also include patient satisfaction or patient response to the health care system (Peabody et al., 2006).

The change in mindset away from apportioning blame and towards a more systems-oriented approach was associated with different technical approaches to the assessment and monitoring of quality of care. Several newer approaches that arose were total quality management (TQM), performance improvement (PI), continuous quality improvement (CQI) and, the most recent approach, quality improvement or QI (Lock, 1994; Institute of Medicine, 2001a; Institute of Medicine, 2001b; Maier and Rhodes, 2001; JHPIEGO, 2008) (Table 1).

The two most recently coined terms Performance Improvement (PI) and Quality Improvement (QI) are often used interchangeably. Both PI and QI assert the need for data and take a systems view. Both PI and QI attempt to avoid attribution of blame and reactive stances, and work to create systems that prevent errors from happening. Results are achieved through a process that considers the institutional context, describes desired performance, identifies gaps between desired and actual performance, identifies root causes, selects interventions to close the gaps, and measures changes in performance. Although many similarities exist between the two processes, the two concepts are subtly different. Quality Improvement (QI) shifts the focus from clinical performances and emphasizes the leading role that systems play as a comparable contributor to outcomes. The notable distinction between the theories of the two processes can be defined as follows: PI implies a particular emphasis on human performance within the system while QI emphasizes the equivalent yet separate contributions of both system and human components. QI processes also emphasize implementation of corrective actions and policy changes (JHPIEGO 2008).

Despite their differences, these processes all have the common goal of improving health care by providing high-quality sustainable health services through measuring and improving institutional and individual outcomes. All of the processes use detailed data to identify areas for improvement, and then formal planned and organized activities are undertaken to ensure that the best possible patient outcomes are achieved.

2.2 Elements of quality improvement

QI is based on structured and continuous evaluations of processes of care and outcomes. Quality management across industries (of which QI in health care is a component) is a complex field based on theories of human motivation, organizational behaviour, research, statistics and evidence-based studies. The hard work and motivation of clinicians, although important, are not enough, and especially not enough to understand and address systems issues (American College of Surgeons, 2006). The goal is to minimize the gap between theory and the realities of implementation. QI methods must be systematically practised within a well designed organizational structure. Morbidity and mortality (M & M) reviews by individual specialties or departments can serve as a foundation for the QI process, but additional processes such as regular multidisciplinary reviews must support a mature QI programme. Examples of particular trauma QI techniques and evidence supporting their use are described in detail in a later section of this book. The focus here is the essential attributes required to establish a formal QI programme.

In general, formal QI programmes must have the essential attributes listed in Table 3. Specifically, the QI process must have authority and be accountable. Clinical care is multidisciplinary, extending across multiple departments and a wide range of hospital staff as well as various physical locations within a hospital. Because of the vast scope of influence mandated by the QI process, the leader, usually a clinician, must be given authority by the hospital (or by appropriate bodies, in the case of QI for region-wide trauma systems). Since multiple disciplines are necessary to achieve optimal patient outcomes and must participate in the QI process, the leader of QI must be held accountable and should be empowered to make administrative decisions – including checking credentials, assessing abilities, and actively participating with others in hospital management in hiring and dismissal decisions for staff involved in patient care. Active participation and buy-in to the formal QI process is required from the medical staff, as well as nursing and administration. For region-wide trauma systems, similar participation and buy-in is required from other stakeholders such as prehospital care providers and those providing rehabilitation services.

In order to be effective, QI must be structured and organized, and must be practised at regular intervals. Objectively defined standards to determine

TABLE 3 **Principles fundamental to the success of a QI programme**

The programme must be scheduled, planned and organized.
There must be a dedicated clinician leader who takes the lead in ensuring quality and is invested with power and authority by the hospital administration (i.e. authority and accountability are essential components of QI).
QI must be multidisciplinary in nature and achieve buy-in from all participants.
Peer review processes must be uniform, nonpolitical and honest, and should incorporate evidence-based medicine.
Evaluations must be critical, but not destructive. A fair and nonpartisan approach that respects the opinions and role of the deliverers of health care is essential.
The programme must be driven by predefined objective criteria and outcome definitions.
Infrastructure, logistical support, and investment are needed to ensure the improvement of quality.
Hard data must be incorporated.
Data collection must be ongoing.
The programme should incorporate methods not only for *identifying* problems, but also for *fixing* problems – often termed "corrective strategies".
The programme should measure what is achieved by the corrective strategies to confirm that they have had their intended effect – often termed "closing the loop".
The programme should be implemented with a commitment for sustained activity and improvement using ongoing data monitoring, data analysis and corrective strategies.

Reference: Maier and Rhodes, 2001

quality of care are necessary, as are explicit definitions of outcomes derived from relevant standards. QI must be supported by appropriate infrastructure and reliable methods of data collection. The goal in data collection and analysis is to obtain consistently valid and objective information identifying "opportunities for improvement". Results of analysis must define corrective strategies. A continuous cycle of monitoring, assessment and management should be performed routinely (Maier and Rhodes, 2001; Performance Improvement Subcommittee of the American College of Surgeons Committee on Trauma, 2002; American College of Surgeons, 2006).

The formulation of corrective strategies or action plans in response to identified "opportunities for improvement" is essential to QI. Corrective "strategies" or "action plans" are structured efforts to improve suboptimal performance that is identified through the QI process. Corrective strategies are basically solutions proposed for fixing a problem or process that may be either case-specific or system-specific. Examples of corrective strategies include guidelines, pathways, protocols, education, peer reviews, monitoring and educational interventions for specific clinical skills, and resource upgrades and enhancements (Table 4). A full discussion of potential corrective strategies, particularly as they relate to trauma QI, can be found in section 4.5. The quality of health care delivery must be seen as reality as well as rhetoric, and must be recognized as having equal importance as the cost of health care delivery. Many of the most useful corrective strategies involve transmission of knowledge rather than costly financial or physical plant investments.

Confirmation and documentation of the impact of corrective actions is commonly termed "closing the loop". In addition to identifying problems and implementing solutions, the QI process is dedicated to ensuring that there are measurable improvements in outcome that can be documented in response to the corrective strategies that are implemented (Performance Improvement Subcommittee of the American College of Surgeons Committee on Trauma, 2002; American College of Surgeons, 2006), (Figure 1).

TABLE 4 **Potential corrective strategies**

Guidelines, pathways, and protocols
- implementation of pre-existing guidelines, pathways, and protocols
- original development
- modification

Targeted education
- rounds
- conferences
- journal clubs
- focused reading
- case presentations
- newsletters
- posters
- videos

Peer review presentations

Action targeted at individual providers (a small component of QI)
- counseling
- further training
- restriction of privileges

Enhancement of resources
- facilities
- equipment
- communication

FIGURE 1 **Closing the loop**

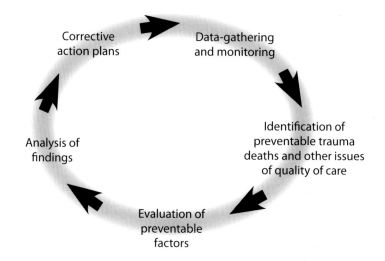

3. Benefits of quality improvement programmes

These guidelines are intended to assist countries to implement trauma QI programmes as a means to lower trauma mortality rates globally, especially in low-income and middle-income countries. Thus, it is appropriate to present the evidence for this recommendation. This section reviews the evidence for the benefits of trauma QI, most of which comes from high-income countries. It also reviews the – thus far – limited reported experience with trauma QI in low-income and middle-income countries. Since such experience is limited, this section also demonstrates the benefits of QI in general in the setting of low-income and middle-income countries – experiences which are eminently transferable to trauma care. Finally, the section comments on the minimal extent of trauma QI programmes globally, pointing out that this is a major deficiency and that the situation could be improved in a low-cost and sustainable manner.

3.1 Review of benefits of trauma quality improvement in the medical literature

In order to ascertain the evidence base that supports the recommendations contained in these guidelines, a review of the published literature on the effectiveness of trauma QI programmes was conducted. A brief summary of the findings of the review are presented here. Details of the review are contained in Annex 1.

The search strategy sought articles that reported on QI programmes or measures that were primarily oriented towards trauma patients. In order for an article to be included, the programme or measure had to have been used to identify correctable deficiencies in patient care, to generate interventions to improve the weakness detected, and to evaluate the implemented solution through measurable outcomes. Articles were not included in the review if they only described QI methodology without evaluating the efficacy of an intervention, if they did not include utilization of QI measures to identify the problem requiring intervention, or if they relied only on subjective evidence such as expert opinion.

A total of 36 articles were identified which fit the search criteria. Most (30) of the articles found discussed QI for trauma patients in the hospital context, while four addressed system-wide QI programmes and two involved the prehospital setting. Thirteen studies evaluated changes in mortality associated with QI, while other patient outcomes (infections, pressure ulcers, and other similar complications) were the main outcome assessed in 12 studies. Process-of-care indicators were the main outcome assessed in 11 studies.

Of the 36 articles reviewed, the vast majority (34) found improvements in mortality, other patient outcomes, or process of care, while only two studies detected no difference after a QI programme or method was implemented. No article reported a worsening of any outcome from a QI programme. Thus, this literature shows that trauma QI programmes consistently improve the process of care, decrease mortality, and improve other patient outcomes. Further efforts to promote trauma QI globally are warranted.

3.2 Experience of trauma quality improvement in low- and middle-income countries

There is a small but growing body of work on trauma QI in low-income and middle-income countries. Some examples are briefly described here. One of the best such reports on the implementation and effectiveness of a QI programme for trauma care comes from the Khon Kaen region of Thailand. This is one of the few such articles that reports on the effect of a QI programme on mortality rates (Box 1).

BOX 1   **Trauma QI programme lowers mortality at Khon Kaen Hospital, Thailand**

Khon Kaen hospital serves a wide rural area in northern Thailand. In order to confront the growing problem of trauma, a trauma registry was set up in the mid-1990s. This indicated a very high rate of potentially preventable deaths. A Trauma Audit Committee reviewed the process of care on expired cases. A variety of problems were found, both in the actions of individual practitioners and in the system. These included difficulties in the referral system, the emergency department, the operating rooms and the intensive care unit. One of the shortcomings found was inadequate resuscitation of patients in shock, both during referral and in the emergency room. Likewise, a high rate of delayed operations for head injuries was also noted. Throughout all of this, there were deficiencies identified in record-keeping and communications among hospital personnel. Corrective action was targeted at the identified problems. This corrective action included: improving communication by radios within the hospital, stationing of fully trained surgeons in the emergency room during peak periods, improving orientation on trauma care for new junior doctors joining the surgery team, and improving the reporting on trauma care through hospital meetings. The trauma registry was able to demonstrate that these improvements increased compliance with medical audit filters (i.e. closing the loop). These changes in process were associated with an improvement in mortality. Overall mortality among admitted trauma cases decreased from 6.1% to 4.4%. These improvements were brought about primarily through improved organization and planning, without high-cost investment in new equipment or infrastructure (Chardbunchachai, Suppachutikul and Santikarn, 2002).

Peer-reviewed preventable death panels have become increasingly used in low-income and middle-income countries. In Pakistan, a peer-reviewed process was employed to identify preventable deaths and potentially preventable deaths in trauma patients admitted over a two-year period. The process revealed possible areas for improvement in system-related factors such as appropriate transfer of patients, treatment delays, inadequate or inappropriate prehospital care, and delay in diagnosis due to equipment malfunction (Jat et al., 2004; Siddiqui, Zafar and Bashir, 2004). A preventable death panel was formed to evaluate all trauma deaths over a 1-year teaching hospital in Tehran. Prolonged prehospital times and deficiencies in resuscitation were found to be largely responsible for the preventable and possibly preventable deaths observed (Zafarghandi, Modaghegh and Roudsari, 2003).

In some low-income and middle-income countries, audits have been used to discern potential low-cost areas of improvement, often when system deficiencies are uncovered by a defining sentinel event. In response to a mass casualty event in 2000, when a hospital in Zimbabwe was overwhelmed by patients injured in a stadium stampede, the hospital's Clinical Audit and Quality Assurance Committee conducted a formal investigation. The report produced by the audit made recommendations for improvement of disaster preparedness that were implemented in multiple contexts, including the prehospital setting, all hospital departments, and the Ministry of Health (Madzimbamuto, 2003).

In South Africa, missed error theory used in aeronautical safety was adapted to analyse missed injuries in trauma patients. These missed injuries were classified according to an established taxonomy of error in order to detect patterns leading to these events. This study revealed three general contexts during which errors leading to missed injuries occurred, namely:

- clinical evaluation;
- radiological assessment;
- surgical exploration.

Errors were classified under these three categories and then further classified by error type:

- "rules-based mistakes" (deviations from well-accepted algorithms);
- "knowledge-based mistakes" (errors made when patients present with an atypical clinical situation and, instead of following an algorithm, the clinician has to rely on his or her problem-solving ability using basic medical principles);
- "errors of execution" (which occur when the correct decisions are made but the execution of the decision is flawed).

The technique of grouping these findings according to the rules of error taxonomy yielded patterns that point to solutions that could be implemented on the systems level (Clarke et al., 2008).

Several countries have reported the use of formal outcome scoring, such as the Trauma and Injury Severity Score (TRISS), in order to detect potentially preventable deaths in their institutions (Boyd, Tolson and Copes, 1987). In Brazil, TRISS scoring was used to monitor the effect of implementation of a regional prehospital programme. This confirmed an increase in triage of the more severely injured to appropriate facilities, which was one of the goals of the programme (Scarpelini, Andrade and Dinis Costa Passos, 2006). In Pakistan, TRISS methodology was used to assess deficiencies in trauma outcomes and uncovered weaknesses in prehospital care. This appraisal resulted in recommendations to decrease the time to arrival in the prehospital care setting and to implement a hospital transfer protocol (Zafar et al., 2002). At a trauma centre in Mumbai, India, TRISS methodology was used to assess outcomes in order to compare their performance with data available from the United States and to identify possible areas for improvement (Goel, Kumar and Bagga, 2004; Murlidhar and Roy, 2004).

Thus there is a growing body of work on the implementation of QI methods for trauma care in low-income and middle-income countries in many areas of the world. The methods are reported to be useful in identifying problems that can be addressed through corrective action. However, so far only a few of these countries have documented improvements in outcome through such corrective action.

3.3 Experience of quality improvement in other fields in low- and middle-income countries

Although there has been limited experience with trauma QI in most low-income and middle-income countries, there has been more experience with QI in other fields. An exhaustive review of the role of QI in health in general is beyond the scope of this publication; however, a few illustrative examples are provided from a range of countries. Many of the examples come from care of medical (rather than surgical) conditions. For instance, in Malawi, an audit of antibiotic usage revealed large-scale inappropriate use and led to implementation of treatment guidelines (Maher, 1996). In Nigeria, the institution of a QI programme in a network of primary health care clinics improved the management of diarrhoea (Zeitz et al., 1993). In rural India, practitioners' skills in paediatric case management were improved through a QI process that involved provision of standard case-management information along with tracking, monitoring and feedback on performance (Chakraborty, D'Souza and Northrup, 2000; Peabody et al., 2006).

There has been some similar progress in fields more directly related to trauma care, including surgery and obstetrics. In Pakistan, Noorani, Ahmed and Esufali (1992) reported on the implementation of a locally-designed low-cost surgical audit system. They demonstrated improved reporting of chest and wound infections, which led to the development of protocols for improved antibiotic prophylaxis. In Malaysia, Inbasegaran, Kandasami and Sivalingam (1998) reported a QI programme involving a two-year audit of 14 hospitals, in which all deaths within seven days of surgery were evaluated by a peer-review process. Areas for improvement were identified and the participating hospitals were informed of the weaknesses detected by the programme in order to carry out improvement measures. In Kuala Lumpur, Malaysia, a similar process carried out for anaesthetic complications in order to identify the root causes of adverse events and to minimize the risk of future similar events (Choy, Lee and Inbasegaran, 1999). More recently, the Thai Royal College of Anesthesiologists has established a multicentred registry to detect adverse events related to peri-operative anaesthetic complications (Boonmak et al., 2005; Punjasawadwong et al., 2007).

Some of the best examples of the role of QI programmes in low-income and middle-income countries come from the field of obstetric care. A specific type of QI for obstetric care is the maternal death audit. This has proved instrumental in improving obstetric care globally (Bhatt, 1989; Mbaruku and Bergstrom, 1995; Ifenne et al., 1997; Pathak et al., 2000; Ronsmans, 2001). Pathak and colleagues demonstrated that the majority of facility-based maternal deaths in Nepal were due to correctable factors, such as delays in treatment at the facilities, inappropriate treatment, and lack of blood (Pathak et al., 2000). In Zaria, Nigeria, it was shown that such QI monitoring assisted with the decrease in time interval between admission and treatment from 3.7 to 1.6 hours (Ifenne et al., 1997). Similar QI related improvements in the process of care led to a decrease in the case fatality for obstetric complications from 12.6% to 3.6% in Kigoma, Tanzania (Mbaruku and Bergstrom, 1995).

A model programme for improving maternal care through QI processes (maternal death audit) in a district hospital in Senegal was based on a daily review of cases by senior specialists in obstetrics and gynaecology. For any maternal death, these senior staff interviewed the staff concerned with the case and the patient's family. Standardized information was obtained and reviewed at weekly meetings. Two senior specialists reviewed the charts of all maternal deaths annually to classify causes of death and contributing factors. This led to detailed recommendations for corrective action. These findings and recommendations were then presented regularly to the audit committee which consisted of staff of the hospital and Ministry of Health, and community representatives. Points for action were agreed on. These actions were then carried out by an executive coordination team (doctors, nurses and other staff) under the supervision of the manager of district health services. Actions included those taken at the district hospital and the network of primary care clinics. Each subsequent year the manager of district health services evaluated how well the recommendations for action had been implemented. The main recommendations focused on improving the 24-hour availability of essential drugs and blood and the availability of basic emergency obstetric care at both hospitals and clinics. Over a four-year period, the case-fatality rate for women delivering at the hospital decreased from 6.0% to 2.6%, primarily due to decreases in deaths due to haemorrhage and hypertensive disorders (Dumont et al., 2006).

The above improvements in emergency obstetric care are directly relevant to efforts to improve trauma care through QI programmes. In both cases, there is a need to arrange capabilities for emergency transport from the field. At health care facilities there is a need for capabilities for resuscitation, including availability of blood, and provision of basic surgical procedures, including both the human resources (skills, staffing) and physical resources (equipment and supplies) to perform these procedures safely. The above examples from obstetric care demonstrate the substantial benefits that can accrue from improvements in organization and planning for services through QI programmes.

Finally, improving the quality of medical care through such measures as QI programmes has been shown by the Disease Control Priorities Project (DCPP) to be very cost-effective. Cost-effectiveness ratios for such efforts range from US$ 4 to US$ 28 per disability adjusted life year (DALY)[2] averted, in circumstances where disease prevalence is high and existing quality of care is low. These cost-effectiveness ratios are in the range of the most cost-effective interventions studied by the DCPP. The cost-effectiveness ratios of interventions studied by the DCPP from US$1 per DALY averted (very cost-effective) to over US$ 20 000 (not cost-effective) (Laxminarayan et al., 2006; Peabody et al., 2006). Moreover, QI programmes themselves can also lead to cost savings. Several of the studies mentioned in section 3.1 directly reported cost savings as one of their outcomes (Civetta, Hudson-Civetta and Ball, 1996; Mathews et al., 1997; Thomas et al., 1997; Collin, 1999; DiRusso et al., 2001).

The DCPP review also concluded that, in efforts to improve the quality of medical care, policies affecting structural conditions (e.g. legal framework, administrative regulations, professional oversight, and the existence of

---

[2] Disability adjusted life year (DALY) is a measure of public health burden of diseases. It takes into account life years lost by subtracting the ages at which people die from various conditions from their life expectancy. It also includes measures of the burden from non-fatal conditions by considering the percentage loss in function. For example, a condition that partially incapacitates someone, leaving them at 50% functional level, results in half of the DALY losses of a fatal condition. Loss from fatal and non-fatal consequences of diseases are then summed for an overall total burden. In a similar fashion, measures of the public health contribution of interventions can be assessed by estimating the numbers of DALY losses that they can avert.

national and local clinical guidelines) were as important as policies that directly addressed the provision of care. These findings are directly in line with the more recent approaches to QI that focus on systems issues and not solely the actions of individual providers (Laxminarayan et al., 2006; Peabody et al., 2006).

The previous three sections have demonstrated that the medical literature strongly supports the role of trauma QI in improving the process and outcome of trauma care. There is a small but growing body of work demonstrating the use of trauma QI in low-income and middle-income countries. Thus far, few of these studies provide outcomes assessments. However, there is a much larger body of work that demonstrates the significant benefit of QI in a variety of other fields in low-income and middle-income countries, much of which, especially for obstetric care, is of direct relevance to trauma care. Moreover, the estimates from DCPP show the significant cost-effectiveness of QI measures in low-income and middle-income countries. All of these considerations demonstrate the important role that trauma QI can have in improving care and outcome for trauma patients globally, especially in low-income and middle-income countries. However, as is shown in the next section, trauma QI programmes are not nearly as well utilized as they could be, in high-income countries and especially in low-income and middle-income countries.

3.4 Status of trauma quality improvement globally

QI programmes are generally regarded as a major foundation of trauma systems in high-income countries. For example, in the United Kingdom, the British Trauma Society mandated that all hospitals caring for major trauma patients should have an audit programme to maintain quality standards in trauma care (Oakley, 1994). In the United States, the American College of Surgeons (ACS) has established criteria that hospitals caring for the injured must meet in order to be designated as various levels of trauma centres. These are laid out in detail in the publication *Resources for optimal care of the injured patient* (American College of Surgeons, 2006). The presence and adequate functioning of a QI programme is a criterion of major importance in trauma centre verification visits by the ACS. Moreover, it is the criterion that is most often found deficient in such visits.

A review of verification visits to 179 hospitals showed that the leading factor associated with unsuccessful review was the absence or deficiencies in QI programmes. The authors of the summary of verification reviews felt that QI programmes were not well understood and that more emphasis on them was needed when developing trauma systems. Examples of the QI deficiencies included failure to correct problems that had been identified, lack of documentation (especially of doctor response times), lack of adherence to protocols, lack of attendance to a regular multidisciplinary QI conference, and lack of utilization of an existing trauma registry to support a QI programme

(Mitchell, Thal and Wolferth, 1994; Mitchell, Thal and Wolferth, 1995). A lack of QI programmes has been found in other high-income countries. Browne et al. (2006) report the results of a survey of 161 hospitals in England, Wales and Northern Ireland that assessed compliance with trauma care standards published by the Royal College of Surgeons and the British Orthopaedic Association. Only 55% of hospitals surveyed had multidisciplinary trauma audit meetings, while 40% of hospitals did not submit trauma data to the Trauma Audit and Research Network (TARN) which is the trauma registry in the United Kingdom (Browne et al., 2006).

Thus, even in high-income countries, there is considerable room for improvement. However, the situation is far more pronounced in low-income and middle-income countries. A study carried out as part of the Essential Trauma Care Project looked at the status of trauma care capabilities at 100 health care facilities in four countries (Ghana, India, Mexico, Viet Nam). In addition to evaluating human and physical resources, this study also looked at the status of administrative mechanisms. Notably, formal trauma-related QI programmes were completely absent, as were trauma registries with adjustment for severity. Moreover, trauma cases were integrated into broader QI programmes in only a minority of circumstances (Table 5) (Mock et al., 2004; Mock et al., 2006). Given this dearth of trauma QI activities in hospitals and trauma systems globally, and given the low cost and potential benefits of such activities for strengthening trauma care, we strongly recommend the upgrading of trauma QI activities globally, whether through formal QI programmes in larger hospitals or by the incorporation of trauma cases into broader QI programmes in smaller facilities.

In attempting to promote greater implementation of trauma QI globally, it is important to note that there are firm foundations to build on. Most large hospitals in which there are surgical and other specialty departments have institutionalized morbidity and mortality (M & M) reviews (see section 4.1), even if these are not part of larger or more in-depth QI activities. A brief summary of the existence and use of M & M conferences is provided in Table 6. A small survey of 16 hospital directors and trauma service directors from seven countries asked about their use of this basic QI technique. The vast majority of these institutions (primarily large, often tertiary care facilities) did have regular departmental meetings at which mortality was discussed. A moderate number of locations engaged in multidisciplinary QI activities. However, very few locations engaged in system-wide trauma QI. Likewise, in only three (of 16) cases were the results of these QI activities reviewed by any outside group (usually the Ministry of Health) (Mock, 2007). Nonetheless, a firm foundation of M & M conferences is present in many large hospitals. The following sections of this book give recommendations about how M & M conferences can be better utilized to identify problems in trauma care and to initiate, direct and monitor

20

corrective action to fix these problems. The book then goes on to discuss how M & M conferences can be built on to establish more formal and more effective trauma QI programmes.

TABLE 5 **Administrative and organizational functions at facilities in four countries**

	Clinic				Small hospital				Large hospital			
	G	**V**	**I**	**M**	**G**	**V**	**I**	**M**	**G**	**V**	**I**	**M**
Trauma-related quality improvement programme	n/a	n/a	n/a	n/a	n/a	n/a	n/a	n/a	0	0	0	0
Trauma cases integrated into broader quality improvement programmes	0	1	0	0	0	2	0	1	1	2	1	1
Trauma registry with severity adjustment	n/a	n/a	n/a	n/a	n/a	n/a	n/a	n/a	0	0	0	0

G: Ghana; **V**: Viet Nam; **I**: India; **M**: Mexico. Compliance with essential trauma care criteria was assessed as: **n/a** (not applicable for that level), **0** (absent), **1** (inadequate), **2** (partly adequate), **3** (adequate).
Source: Table 6 from Mock et al. (2006). Reproduced by kind permission of Springer Science and Business Media.

TABLE 6 **Existence and frequency of morbidity and mortality conferences at 16 institutions in 7 low-income and middle-income countries (Brazil, Colombia, Ghana, Mexico, Romania, Sri Lanka, Viet Nam)**

	Departmental M & M conferences	Multidisciplinary M & M review at institution	Multidisciplinary M & M review for region
Daily	1		
Weekly	5		
Every two weeks	2	1	
Monthly	5	4	1
Every two months		2	
Annually	1		2
Rare / sometimes		3	2
None	2	6	11
TOTAL	16	16	16

Source: Mock, 2007.

4. Techniques of trauma quality improvement

A number of different well defined techniques are used for QI processes. Methods that have been successful for trauma QI include: M & M conferences, panel reviews of preventable deaths, tracking of audit filters (including complications and sentinel events), and statistical methods (including calculation of risk-adjusted mortality rates). This section discusses these major approaches for trauma QI programmes. Detailed descriptions of strategies for potential corrective action to address problems identified by trauma QI methodologies are also reviewed. The section then goes on to discuss application of these methodologies for prehospital and system-wide trauma QI activities and also discusses the role of data sources (medical records and trauma registry) in QI activities. The section finishes with a set of policy recommendations on the appropriateness of different QI techniques at different levels of the health care system.

4.1 Morbidity and mortality (M & M) conferences

M & M conferences (also known as "deaths and complications conferences") involve a discussion of deaths and complications in order to look for preventable factors. M & M conferences are performed around the world in many hospitals – almost everywhere where there are formal medical specialty departments and often in smaller hospitals as well. Trauma cases are frequently included in such M & M conferences, especially in hospitals that have surgery departments. The peer review process involved in the M & M conference is the foundation for improvements in medical care through more formal QI programmes. Typically, all types of cases are discussed at M & M conferences. Likewise, all deaths, complications, adverse events and errors should be discussed. In order to optimize the effectiveness of M & M conferences, the meetings must be viewed not only as discussions of deaths and complications but as opportunities to identify problems. After the conclusion of the M & M conference, clinicians should move forward and take further action to solve the problems that are identified at the conference (Table 7).

M & M conferences should be held at regularly scheduled times, according to the institution's volume of trauma. Hospitals that have higher trauma volumes may have specific M & M conferences on trauma alone, rather than trauma cases being incorporated into the broader departmental M & M conferences. Many hospitals with high trauma volumes hold M & M conferences weekly. However, hospitals with low trauma volumes may have sufficient opportunity to address deaths and complications associated with trauma care on a monthly basis. While the first hour of patient care in trauma has been called "The Golden Hour", the M & M conference has also been dubbed "The Golden Hour" of the surgical working week (Hutter et al., 2006).

Issues related to strengthening M & M conferences are included in Table 7. Readers are also referred to Campbell (1988) for an excellent reference on procedural issues in M & M conferences.

Much better use could be made of M & M conferences for trauma care globally. These conferences are already being conducted in many hospitals – especially those with specialty departments. However, these conferences are often not well utilized to achieve the goals of identifying and correcting problems. Two major improvements could change this. The first is more attention to detail in terms of procedures for conducting the conference (as in Table 7). The other is more attention to detail in identifying problems (especially those relating to systems issues), developing reasonable corrective action plans, following through on implementing these plans, and evaluating whether the corrective action has had its intended consequences. In this regard, section 4.5 on corrective action is as applicable to M & M conferences as it is to any other QI techniques.

Trauma quality improvement committee

A separate multidisciplinary trauma QI committee is an extension of the M & M conference. The trauma QI committee meeting can either be integrated into the departmental M & M conference format or at larger hospitals can be a freestanding meeting. At larger hospitals, the leader of the trauma QI process is often designated by the institution as the "trauma director" and requires adequate administrative support. This administrative support is in the form of a trauma programme manager and trauma programme administrative assistants who are responsible for logistics, data processing, resource allocation, and communication with the complex array of doctors, nurses and supportive services that are involved. Active participation and buy-in to the formal QI process is required from the entire trauma and critical care teams as well as from doctors in other specialties such as anaesthesia, orthopaedics, emergency medicine, neurosurgery, the blood bank (transfusion services) and radiology. Other important contributors to the QI process are administrative and nursing staff from the prehospital arena, the emergency department, intensive care unit (ICU), and operating room.

Support staff who are essential to the infrastructure of QI include the trauma programme manager and trauma registrars (i.e. those who work with the trauma registry) who are responsible for logistics and data collection. Minutes should be taken at the trauma QI committee meeting and should reflect the review, discussion and analysis of the case in question and should also include the proposed corrective action if applicable. Whether for such trauma QI committee proceedings or for departmental M & M conferences, information from discussions is best recorded by means of a standardized form. Such a form can

TABLE 7 **Morbidity and mortality conference FAQ (frequently asked questions)**

Q. When should the meetings be held?
A. Meetings should be held at a time of day chosen with the specific goal of making attendance a dedicated priority. It should be a convenient and regularly scheduled time that accommodates the clinical responsibilities of doctors who attend. Often, this means in the early morning or late afternoon depending on the schedule of the institution. The time for the M & M conference should be protected, and attendance should be mandatory.

Q. How long should the meeting last?
A. Standard educational research shows that adults find it difficult to concentrate when seated in a lecture-type session for longer than 40 minutes. Forty minutes is ideal, though some centres choose 45 minutes or an hour-long session. An important point regarding the length of the session is that it should always be the same. Sessions should start promptly as scheduled and end at the appointed time in order to optimize attendance.

Q. Who should attend the M & M conference?
A. Attending (consultant, fully trained) doctors, resident trainees, and medical students should be required to attend. M & M conferences for trauma are often held in surgery departments. Additionally, other disciplines may be invited to a specific meeting if they were involved in the care of the patient under discussion. Examples of other practitioners who might be invited to attend a trauma M & M periodically are anaesthesiologists, emergency physicians, or general practitioners working in the emergency department, receiving casualty ward, or resuscitation area. Senior nursing staff may also be invited to participate.

Q. Who should lead the meeting?
A. A designated senior or junior doctor who is well respected should lead the meeting. The leader must be a good organizer, must be seen as fair and impartial, and should be able to foster discussion and draw out participants in the conference who may have good contributions to make but who feel uncomfortable when speaking in public. Importantly, the leader must make the meeting a priority and be enthusiastic about the process. If the leader is not committed and enthusiastic, one cannot expect that other members of the group will be.

Q. What should be discussed?
A. The conference should discuss all deaths (operative and non-operative), all complications, quality concerns, and adverse events and errors.

Q. How should patient care issues identified at the meeting be addressed and fixed?
A. The goal of an M & M conference is to discuss and analyse deaths and complications with the goal of learning from the suboptimal outcomes. A productive conference discussion should be able to identify potential areas of improvement in care. An appropriate corrective strategy should then be developed and applied in an effort to optimize care in the future. A process should also be in place to ensure that follow-up takes place to evaluate the effectiveness of the corrective strategies in achieving the goal of improved quality of care (Campbell, 1988).

help to make sure that important information is addressed in the peer review process, including discussion of corrective action. A sample of a QI tracking form is included in Annex 2 (Performance Improvement Subcommittee of the American College of Surgeons Committee on Trauma, 2002; American College of Surgeons, 2006).

On occasion, the trauma QI process identifies an unanticipated poor outcome and in response creates an ad hoc committee with the express goal of formulating a corrective action or specific protocol to improve care from evidence-based guidelines. Unfortunately, because of health care workers' responsibilities and the high demand for their time, these committees are often troublesome to organize and difficult to motivate. In reality, these types of goals are better achieved when incorporated into an existing meeting and already dedicated conference time. The meeting attendees can comprise a working group to review and discuss the evidence and formulate a protocol that is relevant to the institution's needs. It is also much easier to obtain buy-in from practitioners for protocols if the practitioners have played an active role in developing these protocols. Doctors and/or nursing staff who are skilled facilitators who encourage constructive discussion and positive interactions, as well as contributions from team members are essential to make such working groups a success.

4.2 Preventable death panel review

A preventable death panel reviews deaths at either an individual hospital or system, and look for deaths that are considered, by consensus, to have been preventable. Examples of preventable deaths are those resulting from airway obstruction or isolated splenic injuries (i.e. injuries that could be treated successfully in almost any location in the world). Outcome is objective (i.e. death), but designation of a death as preventable is more subjective. In general, panel reviews have been shown to improve system functioning, especially as regards rapid transport, early assessment, appropriate surgical interventions and fewer deaths from preventable causes – especially haemorrhage and airway obstruction. The preventable death panel poses the question: "Is the outcome of death in a particular case definitely preventable, potentially preventable or non-preventable?" The judgement is made by a multidisciplinary panel of experts who assess the care given both by the providers and the system. The preventable death panel decides whether, given optimal care throughout the patient's course, there was any potential to prevent the death, or whether the death was inevitable in view of the severity of the injuries? Even in the best-case scenario would the outcome still be fatal? Although lacking in quantitative precision, these reviews are often a major stimulus for improvements in trauma care (Sanddal, Esposito and Hansen, 1995; Trunkey, 1999; Maier and Rhodes, 2001).

The preventable death panel review was one of the earliest techniques used to assess the development of a trauma system. The method is still one of the simplest and most straightforward techniques and requires minimal resources. Preventable death panel reviews are extremely valuable and have the advantage of not relying on extensive data collection and complex analysis techniques. The goal of a preventable death review is to combine data that are relatively easily accessible in order to assess whether any potential improvements in either the system or the clinical care could prevent mortality.

Data for preventable death studies can come from multiple sources including: the hospital record, prehospital information, highway patrol/traffic safety/police records, death certificates, autopsy reports, and even direct statements or interviews with care providers involved with the case (Sanddal, Esposito and Hansen, 1995; Esposito et al., 1999). This section describes how to undertake a successful preventable death panel review, including: how to constitute a review committee; what information is necessary; how to collect, collate and distribute this information; the specifics of the case review process; and the process of documenting the final discussion and analysis, including suggested corrective actions (Sanddal, Esposito and Hansen, 1995).

Constituting the panel

Important aspects of the case review process include selection and training of the panel, organization, timing and location of the review meeting, judgement criteria for the panel, and record-keeping. All preventable death panels should have a chairperson responsible for leading and organizing the case review process and the meeting. The chairperson must understand all phases of care for the trauma patient, have a broad perspective, remain unbiased, and have the organizational skills to lead the panel through productive discussions that are enthusiastic and probing yet nonconfrontational and productive. The participants should ideally find the meetings enjoyable. Members should maintain an environment of respect as well as honesty regarding the suboptimal outcome of death and must share the common goal of improving future care through the often challenging process of critically assessing each death.

Panel selection needs to be approached thoughtfully. The panel must be multidisciplinary in nature (Table 8). Personnel from all parts of the care process should be represented – including prehospital systems, the various areas of care throughout the hospital such as the emergency department (casualty ward, resuscitation bay), operating room (theatre), and wards. If the reviews are part of an ongoing trauma QI process, the panel should meet routinely, at fixed times and in a neutral setting. Depending on the volume of a hospital or trauma system, the preventable death panel could meet monthly or quarterly. Less often than quarterly is not ideal since regular and more frequent meetings will help

TABLE 8 **Example of preventable death panel participants**

Prehospital provider

Emergency department[1] nurse

Emergency physicians or general doctors involved with trauma patients in emergency department setting

Surgeons involved with trauma care, including (as locally appropriate) general surgeons, orthopaedic surgeons, traumatologists, and others.

Anaesthesiologist

Neurosurgeon, if available

Pathologist or forensic medicine expert/coroner

Radiologist, if there are X-rays or other radiological studies that are related to the case(s) being discussed.

Nursing staff from operating theatre or intensive care unit

[1]Emergency department is also referred to as casualty ward or resuscitation bay in some locations.

to achieve more regular attendance and participation by the panel members – elements that are fundamental for a productive process. Panel members should be selected on the basis of their willingness, commitment and availability to attend the panel reviews. Panel members must see the regular meetings as a priority and must be willing to arrange their often busy schedule so that they can attend and contribute to the process. A multidisciplinary panel has been shown to be extremely beneficial for adequate analysis of data. While some earlier publications state that the inclusion of different disciplines contributes to disagreement, a multidisciplinary panel provides critical information and a fuller perspective of the various aspects of care and is more likely to develop a useful evaluation of the data. In order to accomplish a useful evaluation, the members must have adequate opportunity for discussion. With careful attention to the composition of the panel and appropriate preparation, preventable death panel reviews can achieve levels of agreement approximating to 90% (MacKenzie et al., 1992).

Preparation of data for the review

The chair of the preventable death panel usually reviews all the data sources in advance of the meeting. A wide variety of data sources may be used (Table 9). Normally, the chair or a designated assistant compiles written abstracts summarizing the details of each case. Either the chair or a designated assistant might write a short summary of the case while the assistant should gather data such as the demographics, admission vital signs, and other information that is appropriate or available (e.g. admission Glasgow Coma Scale score, Injury Severity Score, and probability of survival) to include in the abstract. Examples

TABLE 9 **Sources of data for the preventable death panel review**

The hospital record
Overall, a key piece of information. Several key components to be read are:
- emergency department record
- nursing notes
- operative record, including anaesthesia documentation
- radiographic records
- laboratory and blood bank records
- ward and intensive care unit records
- discharge summary

Prehospital information
This is often difficult to obtain but it can be particularly helpful in assessing prehospital vital signs and in documenting the time from injury to hospital arrival and death. Documentation of significant haemodynamic instability or cardiac arrest in the field can clearly add to information suggesting that a trauma death was non-preventable.

Highway patrol/traffic safety/police records
These are especially useful in developing injury prevention measures. Information from local police regarding traffic safety can contribute by identifying areas or situations that might have frequent deaths. Identification of problem areas or intersections where pedestrian or cyclists are injured can often spur simple low-cost improvements focusing on injury prevention.

Autopsy report
Autopsy reports are a rich source of information. Many of the first preventable death studies performed were based solely on autopsy data (West, 1981). As autopsies are expensive and time consuming, many systems and hospitals do not perform them routinely. However, when they are performed, the information from them should be utilized by the panel. Many of the definitely preventable deaths are obvious from autopsy reports (e.g. isolated splenic injury, malpositioned endotracheal tube).

Death certificate
Although a resource, death certificates are often do not contain enough detail to provide the specific information necessary to examine critically why a patient died and whether the death might have been preventable, unless an autopsy report is also included.

Other information such as direct statements or interviews with care providers involved with the case
This verbal source of data is often overlooked but can be extremely helpful. Providers intimately involved in a case will have much knowledge that is not obtainable from written records. An example of information available from a provider's input might be identification of deficiencies not recorded in a chart, such as delays in locating a chest tube in a timely manner in a patient who died secondary to a tension pneumothorax or difficulty in obtaining blood transfusions quickly in patients with large splenic or liver injuries.

Trauma registry data/injury severity data, if available
Although extremely valuable, this data source is very resource-dependent. If available, Injury Severity Score (ISS) and probability of survival (Ps) are particularly useful. (See section 4.4 for more details.)

of components that would be included in a summary abstract can be found in Table 10. The summary abstracts are provided to each panel member. A standardized form can be useful for gathering and summarizing the data and for writing the abstract. A sample data abstraction form is included in Annex 3.

The chair assigns the responsibility for each case to be discussed at the panel review meeting to a panel member who was not directly involved with the care of the particular patient. Assignment to an uninvolved panel member

TABLE 10 **Abstract components for summary of preventable death panel review**

Demographics
Mechanism of injury
Transfer status
Mode of arrival
Prehospital/field vital signs (specify exact times)
Vital signs on arrival to emergency department (specify exact time)
Glasgow Coma Scale score on admission
Procedures performed (including advanced airway management such as endotracheal intubation, and operations)

Key time variables
  • estimated time of injury
  • time until arrival at scene of prehospital care providers
  • time of arrival to hospital
  • time until transfusion
  • time of general surgical evaluation
  • time until disposition to operating room, intensive care unit, or ward, and time to death

Injury Severity Score (if available)[1]
Probability of survival (Ps) (if available)[1]

[1]More details on these parameters are given in section 4.4.
Reference: MacKenzie et al., 1992

is essential so that he or she can present an unbiased picture of the events and records. The designated panel member reviews the summary abstract and all the relevant data sources in advance and is responsible for presenting the case and data relevant to it to the full panel at the meeting. Members of the panel responsible for reviewing and presenting a patient chart at the meeting should be provided with copies of the summary abstract and a full copy of the relevant data sources to be reviewed at least one week in advance of the scheduled meeting.

While the panel member designated to review the patient's records in detail and present the relevant data to the panel is provided with more comprehensive data, the remainder of the panel members usually only have the summary for review. In cases where particular components of the chart provide particularly interesting information relevant to the case, copies of those data may be attached to the summary abstract handed out to all panel members. For example, the prehospital information sheet might be provided on a patient with prolonged transport to the hospital, or the emergency department data flowsheet might be provided on a patient who on arrival at the hospital was hypotensive secondary to a splenic injury but was taken to the operating room in a delayed manner.

In addition, it is helpful but not mandatory to provide each panel member with a structured case review form on which they can indicate whether components of each aspect of care are felt to be adequate and timely. In order to maintain confidentiality surrounding the patient's information and in an effort to keep the written documents as anonymous as possible, specific identifying data such name and/or hospital record number are deleted from all the documents distributed. A code number or other means of keeping track of the case can be assigned to the paperwork rather than patient-specific information. A sample case review form is included in Annex 3 and sample abstracts are in Annex 4.

Specifics of the case review process

Panel members should receive a formal orientation during which expectations are set. The designated panel members responsible for presenting cases at the time of the panel meeting should receive full copies of the de-identified data sources at least one week in advance of the scheduled meeting. The chair leads the meeting and guides the discussion and the decision process for determining whether the death was (1) preventable, (2) potentially preventable, (3) non-preventable, or (4) non-preventable but with care that could have been improved. The last item may also help to identify opportunities for improvement in the system, even if the particular death in question could not have been avoided. See Table 11 for full definitions of these terms.

For simplicity, some panels use only three categories (preventable, potentially preventable, and non-preventable) and do not create a separate fourth category for non-preventable deaths in which care could have been improved. Nonetheless, even when deaths are deemed non-preventable, it is best for panels to continue to identify problems in care and to use this information in the development of corrective action plans. This is true whether one or two categories for non-preventable deaths are used. Using the full four categories (including non-preventable but with care that could have been improved) is optimal and requires only minimal extra work compared with using three categories.

Whatever classification system for preventability is used, it must be clearly communicated to the panel members. A standardized case review form to assist the members in keeping track of their critique is useful although not mandatory. See Annex 3 for an example of a standardized case review form. See also Annex 4 for sample abstracts with case-by-case discussions of determination of preventability and corrective action plans. Examples are included from each of the four categories of preventability discussed above.

During the panel discussions, each panel member assigned to a patient presents a summary of the case as well as their analysis of the case to the entire committee. After a discussion, with contributions requested from the

TABLE 11 **Definitions of preventability for death panel review**

1. **Preventable**
   - injuries and sequelae considered survivable;
   - death could have been prevented if appropriate steps had been taken;
   - frank deviations from standard of care that, directly or indirectly, caused patient's death;
   - statistically, probability of survival greater than 50%, or Injury Severity Score (ISS) below 20.[1]

2. **Potentially preventable**
   - injuries and sequelae severe but survivable;
   - death potentially could have been prevented if appropriate steps had been taken;
   - evaluation and management generally appropriate;
   - some deviations from standard of care that may, directly or indirectly, have been implicated in patient's death;
   - statistically, probability of survival 25–50% or ISS between 20 and 50.[1]

3. **Non-preventable**
   - injuries and sequelae non-survivable even with optimal management;
   - evaluation and management appropriate according to accepted standards;
   - if patient had co-morbid factors, these were major contributors to death;
   - statistically, probability of survival less than 25% or ISS above 50.[1]

4. **Non-preventable, but with care that could have been improved**
   - as with non-preventable above, but care is questionable or clear errors in care are detected, even though these did not lead to the death.

---

[1] Probabilities of survival and ISS are meant to be a general guide to classification of preventability of death, not rigid cut-offs. Furthermore, neither probability of survival nor ISS is required for determination of preventability. Many panel reviews are conducted without this information. Additional information on calculation of probability of survival and ISS are found in section 4.4.
References: Sanddal, Esposito and Hansen, 1995; Jat et al., 2004; American College of Surgeons, 2006

entire committee guided by the chair, a vote on the preventability status of the death is taken. One school of thought suggests that the vote should be taken in an open fashion so that members can discuss why they decided on a specific classification and to promote optimal discussion in order to achieve a thorough analysis and consensus. Other chairs and committees feel that ballots should be cast in confidence to avoid peer pressure and hurt feelings if care providers are in the room. This decision must take into account the composition of the preventable death panel as well as potential cultural and political implications of closed or open voting.

Inclusion of involved care providers on the panel: potential for bias

There are two philosophies regarding the participation of doctors or other care providers who were directly involved with a particular patient's care. One theory is that the provider involved in taking care of a patient who died should not participate in the panel. This is based on the concern that the presence of that provider may suppress productive conversations and critical analysis of a case and therefore introduce bias into the ultimate judgement as to whether a death was preventable or non-preventable.

A second theory supports the active participation of a provider involved in the care of the patient. The involved provider must be treated with respect. That provider may often be able to supply information critical to understanding a mortality event and may assist in identifying areas for improvement that might not be recognized otherwise.

The decision whether to include or exclude a practitioner must be made by the preventable death panel chair and will often be based on the culture of a hospital or environment and the number of clinicians who are knowledgeable and able to contribute to critical review of a trauma death. In smaller hospitals, the limited number of staff available may require that all providers, involved or not involved with a trauma patient's care, should participate in the discussion. Whoever attends, it is clear that the critical chart and data review should not be assigned to the treating provider. An objective chart reviewer is essential for discerning the most pertinent and reliable information on the specifics of a patient's care. Although, a treating clinician can be involved in the discussion of the facts, he or she should not be assigned the responsibility of collecting and presenting the facts to the panel.

Preventable death panels: documentation of discussion and analysis

Adequate records of the patient data and the abstract provided to the panelists must be kept. Minutes documenting the panel discussion should also be recorded. At the conclusion of the discussion, the panel chair should be responsible for filling out a summary form detailing the panel discussion and decision. An example of a form that the chair can use to document the final decision of the panel can be found in Annex 3. Potential deficiencies to consider and document can be found in Table 12. Additionally, the potential errors reviewed in section 4.3 should be looked for, and corrective strategies (section 4.5) identified. Any recommendations to improve care, as well as communications with an outside agency, should be documented. For example, if an ambulance service brought a severely injured patient to a small clinic where the patient waited for hours prior to being transferred to a major hospital, an area for improvement is identified. The panel chair might suggest the corrective action of educating the ambulance providers and implementation of a formal policy to take injured patients only to a specific larger hospital rather than to small clinics. A formal letter that suggests this policy could be written by the chair and would serve as documentation of efforts to improve prehospital care.

Preventable death panels: a summary

In conclusion, preventable death panels are a versatile and widely applicable method of trauma QI. They represent the next step beyond the M & M conference. Preventable death panels do have their limitations. One-time or

TABLE 12 **Classification of types and sites of deficiencies**

Possible deficiencies to consider include:
- airway
- haemorrhage control
- chest
- fluid resuscitation
- delays in treatment
- other
- documentation.

Locations of deficiencies to consider include:
- prehospital
- emergency department (ED)
- operating room (OR)
- intensive care unit (ICU)
- ward
- interfacility transfer
- system inadequacy.

References: O'Leary, 1995; Sanddal, Esposito and Hansen, 1995

even intermittent preventable death panels should not be seen as a substitute for a formal trauma QI process. They should be viewed as an extension of the standard M & M process rather than as a replacement for it. Preventable death panels focus on determination of preventability and are often not positioned to make judgements on complex aspects of patient care. The assessment of preventability often depends on the resources and capabilities of an institution and/or system. Although preventability judgements may be viewed as somewhat subjective and there may be variation in reliability between different panels' assessments, death panel reviews nonetheless remain a straightforward method of accomplishing the goal of assessing and improving the quality of care.

Preventable death panel reviews are applicable anywhere in the world, in countries at all economic levels and in both hospital and system-wide settings. The basic materials for a successful preventable death panel are available in any setting that cares for patients. The commitment of enthusiastic and intelligent panel members, the timely distribution of data sources reflecting a patient's course (as described in Table 9), and an interactive discussion by the panel members can assure the success of the panel. Ultimately, preventable death panels have the capacity to identify potential areas of improvement for future patient care which would otherwise not have been identified.

4.3 Tracking of audit filters, complications, errors, adverse events, and sentinel events

The goal of all QI methods is to identify and correct problems. The last two methods described – M & M conferences and preventable death panels – are mostly retrospective in nature with qualitative and sometimes subjective judgements based on chart review, discussion and expert opinion. The next sections (4.3 and 4.4) represent more objective and analytic approaches that utilize prospective data collection. The techniques in this section have in common monitoring for problems and specific events. These events may or may not contribute to unwanted outcomes. Often, these techniques require more extensive resources – such as staff time for data-gathering and computerized information systems.

Audit filters

Audit filters are pre-identified variables that are routinely tracked to identify whether accepted standards of care are being met. Complications, adverse events and errors are examples of many possible types of audit filters. Audit filters can identify issues that may contribute to various complications, including but not limited to death, and also may identify "near misses" in patient care that do not result in a poor outcome but might indicate a patient care process that can be improved. Particular cases identified by the audit filters are then reviewed on a systematic basis to see if indeed there was a problem with the quality of care delivered (Shackford et al., 1987).

A list of potential audit filters that have been screened for in QI programmes is given in Table 13. Some of the most significant audit filters are: patients with abdominal injuries and hypotension who do not undergo laparotomy within one hour of arrival to the emergency department; patients with epidural or subdural haematoma who do not undergo a craniotomy within four hours after arrival at an emergency department; and patients with greater than eight hours between arrival and debridement of an open fracture.

All audit filters can be screened for routinely, or one may screen only for specific filters that have been determined to be of interest to an institution. Audit filters can be broken down into areas of care. Prehospital issues may include appropriate personnel, stabilization, and rapidity of transport. Emergency department issues may include proper utilization of resuscitation principles, protection of airway, intravenous access and resuscitation, and the rapid and complete identification of injuries.

Another important phase captured by audit filters is time to the operating room for various injuries – penetrating abdominal trauma, intracranial mass lesion drainage, and washout and repair of open fracture. Another category is the timely presence of appropriate personnel, such as nursing, medical and

TABLE 13 **Potential audit filters**

Prehospital care
- field scene time >20 minutes;
- missing emergency medical services (EMS) report or absence of prehospital essential data items on EMS report;
- appropriateness of triage and transfer processes.

Emergency department
- timely response of required personnel and resources in attending to patient needs (e.g. response time of surgeons, availability of operating room);
- absence of sequential neurological documentation in the emergency department of trauma patients with a diagnosis of skull fracture, intracranial injury or spinal cord injury;
- absence of at least hourly determination and recording of blood pressure, pulse, respirations, temperature, Glasgow Coma Scale (GCS) score and intake and output (I & O) measurements for a major or severe trauma patient, beginning with arrival in the resuscitation area and including time spent in radiology up to admission to the operating room or ICU, death, or transfer to another hospital;
- lack of documentation of a history and physical examination note by doctor;
- Glasgow Coma Scale score <13 and no head computerized tomography (CT) scan within 2 hours of arrival at hospital (if CT available in hospital);
- Glasgow Coma Scale score <8 and no endotracheal tube or surgical airway performed before leaving resuscitation area.

Time to operating room
- patient with abdominal injuries and hypotension (systolic BP <90) who does not undergo laparotomy within 1 hour of arrival at the hospital;
- delay in performing laparotomy (from greater than 4 hours to greater than 24 hours after admission depending on hospital practice);
- craniotomy after 4 hours, for drainage of epidural or subdural haematoma;
- abdominal, thoracic, vascular or cranial surgery after 24 hours;
- unplanned return to operating theatre within 48 hours of initial procedure.

Other
- patient requiring re-intubation of the airway within 48 hours of extubation;
- non-operative treatment of gunshot wound to the abdomen;
- non-fixation of femoral fracture in adult;
- all delays in identification of injuries;
- all trauma deaths (particularly can focus on unexpected deaths such as those occurring with low Injury Severity Scores);
- required equipment, shared with other departments (e.g. fluid warmer, ventilator), not immediately available when requested;
- sentinel events (see details in next section)
- non-compliance with institutional protocols;
- any case referred by provider (doctor, nurse, or other) for care concerns;
- all major complications (e.g. deep venous thrombosis, pulmonary embolus, decubitus ulcers. See list of potential complications in Table 14).

It is to be emphasized that this is a list of *potential filters*. Specific ones may or may not be useful in a given location, depending on local circumstances.

Reference: Maier and Rhodes, 2001

subspecialty services, as applicable. The various audit filters capture a number of additional concerns such as unplanned operations, delays in care and documentation issues (Copes et al., 1995; American College of Surgeons, 2006).

Audit filters can be approached as either sentinel events or as rate-based filters. Sentinel events are filters for which even one case prompts review, such as death with low Injury Severity Scores (see below for more details on sentinel events). Rate-based filters are those in which a certain low percentage of noncompliance is expected – such as delays in reaching the operating room in patients with open fractures, a certain proportion of whom would be expected to have such delays for valid reasons, such as when care of life-threatening injuries takes precedence. Review is prompted if these filters exceed certain threshold percentages.

Usefulness of audit filters

In high-income countries there recently has been debate on the usefulness of audit filters in trauma QI (Copes et al., 1995; Cryer et al., 1996). Important publications support specific audit filters for both trauma care and prehospital care. Evaluation of 22 filters in the Pennsylvania trauma system identified nine that were useful in identifying patients with a significantly increased risk of mortality or prolonged length of stay in hospital or ICU. Additionally, filters screening for documentation deficiencies identified such deficiencies as being among the most common problems in the process of care (Copes et al., 1995). Specifically focusing on potential audit filters for prehospital trauma care, Rosengart, Nathens and Schiff (2007) evaluated 81 filters and recommended screening for 28 specific prehospital filters. Alternatively, some publications also report audit filters to be useful in identifying documentation deficiencies but not in providing useful information in the quality improvement process (Cryer et al., 1996).

Potential drawbacks of audit filters are the cost and lack of extensive published examples documenting the utility of specific filters. The staff time required and the cost of evaluating audit filters for every trauma patient may prove prohibitive to routine screening for many of the audit filters. As a result, in one particular high-income country (USA), the American College of Surgeons has recently changed from giving a list of specific filters for which trauma QI programmes should audit to merely recommending that QI programmes should track some filters, depending on local priorities (American College of Surgeons, 2006).

However, there is also recent evidence of significant potential benefit of screening for audit filters in several low-income and middle-income countries. One might thus infer that they have greater potential use in circumstances where there are fewer pre-existing trauma QI activities in general. For example, the previously noted trauma QI programme in Khon Kaen, Thailand, tracked 32 audit filters. These were felt to be an important component of the programme's success in reducing preventable deaths (Chadbunchachai et al., 2001; Chadbunchachai et al., 2003). Similar early experience has been reported from Pakistan (Jat et al., 2004).

Alternatively, another way to utilize audit filters is as an adjunct to the preventable death panel review process. Assessing for the defined audit filters during preventable death panel reviews has been shown to identify different types of issues according to the system examined. While assessing preventable deaths in a mature trauma system, the most likely contributors to poor outcomes were delays in treatment and judgement errors (Teixeira et al., 2007). In contrast, in low-income and middle-income countries with a less mature system, different factors were identified as responsible for preventable deaths – including inadequate prehospital care, inappropriate transfer, limited hospital resources, and an absence of integrated trauma care (Jat et al., 2004). Depending on the resources of a hospital or system, consideration should be given to tracking audit filters on every patient who is admitted or, alternatively, audit filters can be used as additional points of analysis in preventable death panel reviews. Likewise, some of the most potentially useful filters to track are complications and errors, as discussed in the next sections.

Complications, adverse events, errors, and sentinel events

Complications are unexpected, unplanned and unwanted outcomes such as a wound infection or a deep venous thrombosis. Complications may be secondary to natural disease processes. Alternatively, complications may result from an adverse event. An adverse event is defined as "an injury that is caused by medical management rather than the underlying disease and that prolongs hospitalization, produces a disability at discharge, or both" (Institute of Medicine, 2001a). While all adverse events are complications, not all complications are secondary to adverse events. A long list of potential complications may be systematically screened for, identified, recorded and tracked as indicators of the quality of care (Table 14).

The process of tracking complications looks for rates of complications that are higher than would normally be expected. If a high rate of a particular complication is identified by the screening and tracking process, a directed investigation should be undertaken to sort out the underlying reasons for the detected increase. Once reasons for the unusual increase in complication rates are identified, corrective measures and strategies should be implemented to reduce the complication rate to an acceptable level.

An error is defined as "failure of a planned action to be completed as intended or use of a wrong plan to achieve an aim" (Institute of Medicine, 1999). An error

TABLE 14 **Potential complications to be tracked**

- Acute Respiratory Distress Syndrome (ARDS)
- Aspiration pneumonia
- Bacteraemia
- Cardiac arrest
- Coagulopathy
- Compartment syndromes
- Dehiscence/evisceration
- Empyema
- Esophageal intubation
- Hypothermia
- Mortality
- Myocardial infarction
- Pneumonia
- Pneumothorax
- Skin breakdown
- Surgical site infection (deep)
- Renal failure
- Urinary track infection
- Unplanned reoperation
- Wound infection
- Deep venous thrombosis/pulmonary embolus

References: Maier and Rhodes, 2001; American College of Surgeons, 2006

can also be thought of as failure to follow accepted practice at an individual or systems level (Edmonds, 2004). An error can result in a poor outcome but an error may also occur without causing any negative impact on outcome. In contrast to a complication or an adverse event, which are by definition end results, an error is a contributing factor. An error that does not result in a bad outcome can also be thought of as a "near miss" (Table 15). While an adverse event can be due to error, most adverse events are not errors. An adverse event attributable to error is a "preventable adverse event".

A particularly egregious adverse event is termed a "sentinel event". A sentinel event is defined as "an unexpected occurrence resulting in death or serious physical or psychological injury, or the risk thereof" (JCAHO, 2005). While all sentinel events are adverse events, not all adverse events are sentinel events. A sentinel event is a severe adverse event with a particularly bad outcome that prompts an immediate and thorough investigation of the circumstances contributing to the poor outcome. When such a bad outcome occurs, a separate QI investigation process called "root cause analysis" (RCA) might be undertaken. RCA is a process for identifying the etiology of the unanticipated poor outcome. The RCA type of QI investigation consists of forming a separate team to analyse the reasons for the poor outcome in a particular case (JCAHO, 2005).

The RCA team should be interdisciplinary and focused on brainstorming to identify and understand unforeseen and unanticipated issues that resulted in the poor outcome. The investigation should be short-lived with quick deadlines.

It is a one-time process that looks at the events behind a particular case rather than an ongoing data collection and data monitoring of all cases. The goal of an RCA team is to analyse thoroughly an unusual event, delineate what care and systems issues allowed such a severe adverse event to occur, and design measures to prevent similar poor outcomes in the future. Although a full discourse on sentinel events and RCA is beyond the scope of this publication, the steps that an RCA uses to address a sentinel event can be a useful guideline in approaching any adverse event that a QI programme might encounter and wish to investigate. Full books and publications describing the complex RCA process in detail can be accessed (Wilson, Dell and Anderson, 1993; Spath, 1997; Ammerman, 1998; JCAHO, 2005; Australian Commission on Safety and Quality in Health Care, 2007).

TABLE 15 **Taxonomy of adverse events and errors**

	ADVERSE EVENT = YES	**ADVERSE EVENT = NO**
ERROR =YES	**PROBLEM** Discuss at department M & M and report to QI committee **QI score** **3** = adverse effect, not life-threatening **4** = physical effect, potentially life-threatening **5** = life-threatening or death	**NEAR MISS** Report to QI committee and discuss as an "opportunity for improvement" **QI score** **1** = unlikely to have adverse effect **2** = potential to have adverse effect
ERROR =NO	May review at M & M and decide that a different treatment may have led to improved outcome, but standard of care was met or a different treatment would not have changed the outcome **QI score** **0** = no evident concerns about quality of care	**NO PROBLEM** **NO ERRORS, NO ADVERSE EVENTS** What we are always trying to achieve

ERROR SCORING

Definition of an error
A. The failure of a planned action to be completed as intended (i.e. error of execution) or the use of a wrong plan to achieve an aim (i.e. error of planning).
B. Treatment that did not meet the standard of care.

Levels of concern
Level 0 = no evident concerns about quality of care.
Level 1 = quality concern that did not affect the patient's well-being and was unlikely to cause an adverse effect on the patient.
Level 2 = quality concern that did not affect the patient's well-being but had the potential to cause an adverse effect on the patient.
Level 3 = quality concern that had an adverse effect but was not life-threatening.
Level 4 = quality concern that caused a major permanent physical effect or was potentially life-threatening.
Level 5 = quality concern that was life-threatening.

References: Institute of Medicine, 1999; Maier and Rhodes, 2001

Classification of errors

Error can be categorized into subtypes. Several taxonomies of types of errors are in use. For example, section 3.2 includes the experience in South Africa of adapting the error theory used in aeronautical safety to trauma QI work. Another useful taxonomy is that developed by the JCAHO (Joint Commission on the Accreditation of Healthcare Organizations) in the USA (Reason, 1995; Chang et al., 2005; Gruen et al., 2006; Ivatury et al., 2008). This classifies errors based on:

- *Impact*: implies the harm done by the error, ranging from none to permanent impairment or death, as delineated in Table 15.
- *Type*: implies the patient care processes that were faulty, such as errors in diagnosis, treatment, prevention, communication and equipment failures.
- *Domain*: implies the setting in which the error occurred, such as prehospital, initial assessment, secondary survey, resuscitation errors, operative errors and critical care errors. Floor ward and rehabilitation errors also occur but are less frequent.
- *Cause*: implies the factors leading to an error. These are usually further grouped into:
  - •• *system errors* that include errors in design, organization and maintenance of both the physical system (e.g. facilities, equipment, infrastructure) and the organizational system (e.g. management, organizational culture, protocols/processes, training);
  - •• *human errors* that involve direct contact with the patient and that are often the proximate cause of the error (A more detailed classification of human errors looks at the process of decision-making and implementation of a management plan in the care of an injured patient. This classifies potential errors as diagnostic, or input, errors, intention errors and execution errors). (See Table 16).

A summary of the terms and definitions of events that could be useful for the QI process to monitor, record and track are included in Table 17.

4.4 Statistical methods: risk-adjusted mortality

A number of different scoring systems exist to help compare injuries between patients in an objective manner. Some of these scoring systems are based on the anatomical nature of the injuries sustained (anatomical scores) and some are based on the physiological status of the patient (physiological scores). The best known and most widely used scoring systems are the Abbreviated Injury Scale (AIS), the Injury Severity Score (ISS), the Glasgow Coma Scale (GCS), the Revised Trauma Score (RTS), the Trauma and Injury and Severity Score (TRISS), and A Severity Characterization of Trauma (ASCOT) (Baker, 1974; Champion, 1989; O'Keefe and Jurkovich, 2001; Association for the Advancement of Automotive

TABLE 16 **Causes of errors**

Diagnostic error
Data are incorrectly perceived.
As a result, an incorrect intention is formulated and therefore the wrong action is performed.

Example: Failure to diagnose intra-abdominal haemorrhage, and subsequent delay in operative intervention.

Intention error
Data are correctly perceived.
Incorrect intention is nonetheless developed and therefore the wrong action is performed.

Example: Awareness of a threatened airway in a hypoxic, head-injured patient, but failure to take steps to clear and establish a secure airway.

Execution error
Data are correctly perceived.
Correct intention is developed.
Wrong or unintended action is performed.

Example: Making the decision to secure the airway with endotracheal intubation, but misplacing the tube in the oesophagus rather than the trachea.

References: Reason, 1995; Chang et al., 2005; Gruen et al., 2006; Ivatury et al., 2008

TABLE 17 **Summary of terms and definitions of events to be monitored, recorded, and tracked**

Term	Definition
Complication	Unexpected, unplanned and unwanted outcomes such as a wound infection or a deep venous thrombosis. Can be secondary to natural disease processes or an adverse event.
Adverse event	"An injury that is caused by medical management rather than the underlying disease and that prolongs hospitalization, produces a disability at discharge, or both." (Institute of Medicine, 2001a)
Error	"Failure of a planned action to be completed as intended or use of a wrong plan to achieve an aim" (Institute of Medicine, 1999)
Sentinel event	A subtype of adverse event with a particularly high potential for harm. "An unexpected occurrence resulting in death or serious physical or psychological injury, or the risk thereof." (JCAHO, 2005)
Audit filters	Pre-identified standards that are routinely tracked and flagged if particular criteria for accepted standards of care are not met. Any of the preceding items in this table may also be used as audit filters.

Medicine, 2005). A detailed comparison of the scoring systems can be found in Table 18.

Through such statistical processes, hospitals evaluate the percentage of deaths occurring in patients with low Injury Severity Scores or a low probability of death based on either one score (e.g. ISS) or on a combination of scores such as the ISS and RTS (TRISS methodology) (Boyd, Tolson and Copes, 1987).

Additionally, a trauma QI programme can set up a system to evaluate unexpected deaths identified by the various scoring systems. For example, the trauma QI programme can mandate examination of all deaths in patients with minor injuries as identified by an ISS of less than 9 or with probability of survival (Ps) greater than 90% as calculated by TRISS to make sure that an appropriate level of care was achieved.

Use of statistical methods also allows a hospital to compare itself against predetermined national or international norms. Hospitals with risk-adjusted death rates higher than expected may warrant evaluation of individual unexpected deaths along with evaluation of the systems of care in order to identify elements that may contribute to such higher risk-adjusted mortality.

Any of the above-noted risk-adjustment methods add increased objectivity to the QI process. However, it must be noted that they also increase resource requirements, especially in terms of staff time for injury severity coding.

TABLE 18 **Scoring system for severity of injury**

System	Definition
Abbreviated Injury Scale (AIS)	Anatomical score. The purpose of the AIS was to catalogue anatomical injuries sustained in motor vehicle collisions. It was developed in 1971 and revised in 1990 by the Association for the Advancement of Automotive Medicine, the American Medical Association and the Society of Automotive Engineers. Injuries are designated according to six body areas and are ranked on a scale from AIS 1 (least severe) to AIS 6 (most severe).
Injury Severity Score (ISS)	Anatomical score. This was developed in 1974 and revised in 1997 (the New ISS, or NISS). It utilizes the AIS system to create a summary score. The ISS is derived from the sum of the squares of the highest AIS scores from each of up to three body regions. ISS can range from 1 to 75 and reflects the likelihood of mortality. A common perspective is that ISS less than or equal to 9 represents a minor injury, from 10-24 is considered a moderate combination of injuries, and greater than 24 represents a severely injured patient. ISS is used to quantify injury objectively and also to assist in estimating the likelihood of survival.
Glasgow Coma Scale (GCS)	Physiological score. Reported in 1970 from Glasgow, Scotland, the GCS is an objective estimate of central nervous system function according to level of consciousness. GCS is based on valuations of the functions of motor response, verbal response, and eye-opening. Scores range from 3 to 15. It is simple and reproducible with low variability but is limited to use in patients with head injury.

Revised Trauma Score (RTS)	Physiological score. This expands physiological scoring from isolated head injury, as reflected by GCS, to a patient's overall physiological status. It incorporates central nervous system function, plus functional status of the respiratory and circulatory systems. It is based on GCS, systolic blood pressure and respiratory rate.
Trauma and Injury Severity Score (TRISS)	Physiological and anatomical score. A method used to assign the probability of survival (Ps) to an individual patient after injury, this is based on a combination of RTS, ISS, mechanism of injury (blunt versus penetrating), and age. Limitations exist, but overall it is an objective measure of the likelihood of survival. TRISS is often used to assign a correlating calculated probability of survival for each patient, ranging from 0-100%.[1]
A Severity Characterization Of Trauma (ASCOT)	Physiological and anatomical score. Developed to address the limitations of TRISS, this uses a more complete set of data. While TRISS has three major predicting variables, ASCOT uses seven predicting variables to calculate a probability of survival. Although it is an attempt to improve the reliability of TRISS, ASCOT is not as widely used because of the complexity associated with collecting the data and calculating ASCOT.

[1] Ps may be calculated by the following formula: $Ps = 1/(1 + e^{-b})$, where $b = b_0 + b_1(RTS) + b_2(ISS) + b_3(A)$. e is the base of the natural logarithm: 2.71828. RTS is the revised trauma score, ISS the Injury Severity Score, and A is a variable for age (0 for age <55, 1 for >55). $b_0 – b_3$ are coefficients derived from using the reference databases that contain large numbers of patients from multiple institutions and thus are considered as norms against which individual patients and individual institutions can be compared.

The most extensively utilized database has been the MTOS (Major Trauma Outcome Study, from the USA in the 1980s), from which the following coefficients were derived: Blunt trauma: $b_0 = -1.2470$; $b_1(RTS) = 0.9544$; $b_2(ISS) = -0.0768$; $b_3(age) = -1.9052$; Penetrating trauma: $b_0 = -0.6029$; $b_1(RTS) = 1.1430$; $b_2(ISS) = -0.1516$; $b_3(age) = -2.6676$.

The above figures were used extensively in calculation of Ps for research and QI work. The above figures are somewhat outdated, but are provided for completeness, as they have been heavily utilized in the literature. They were updated several years later to reflect recalibration based on updated AIS-90 coding: Blunt trauma: $b_0 = -0.4499$; $b_1(RTS) = 0.8085$; $b_2(ISS) = -0.0835$; $b_3(age) = -1.7430$; Penetrating trauma: $b_0 = -2.5355$; $b_1(RTS) = 0.9934$; $b_2(ISS) = -0.0651$; $b_3(age) = -1.1360$.

Data from the MTOS are now 20 years old. A newer reference database, the National Trauma Data Bank of the American College of Surgeons, has been developed. It is anticipated that a newer risk-adjustment model for calculating Ps based on this database will be developed in the following few years and that this will supersede the above-noted TRISS/MTOS method.

References: Baker, 1974; Boyd, Tolson and Copes., 1987; Champion, 1989; Champion et al., 1990; Champion, Sacco and Copes, 1995; Association for the Advancement of Automotive Medicine, 2005; American College of Surgeons, 2009

4.5 Corrective strategies and closing the loop

As described in section 2.2, an essential foundation of a successful QI programme is to develop and institute corrective strategies to address the problems identified, and then to evaluate and document the effectiveness of these strategies. Definitions and examples of some of the main corrective strategies utilized are given below.

Guidelines, pathways, and protocols

Guidelines are defined as systematically developed consensus statements that are designed to assist in clinical decision-making and that usually focus on diagnosis and treatment (Performance Improvement Subcommittee of the American College of Surgeons Committee on Trauma, 2002). Guidelines are usually general in nature and often rated by the power of evidence. Guidelines are commonly developed by societies for surgical, trauma and critical care with the goal of education and dispersing knowledge on the subject of appropriate care. Published practice guidelines provide evidence-based documents from which institution-specific pathways and protocols can be developed.

Pathways and protocols expand on practice guidelines and are used as bedside instruments to influence care. The goal of both pathways and protocols is to decrease treatment variation in clinical management. Protocols are often institution-specific and consist of a step-by-step delineation of procedures for solving a problem or accomplishing a desired outcome. Protocols are often displayed in an algorithm format. While a pathway implies continuous data collection and monitoring, protocols may or may not include a continuous monitoring and data-evaluation component. An example of a protocol specific to trauma would be a "massive transfusion protocol". In order to decrease the variability in the ratio of red blood cells transfused to the volume of clotting factors transfused, a massive transfusion protocol can be designed on the basis of existing data regarding best practices and used as a bedside tool to guide blood product administration in haemorrhaging patients.

Several examples of instituting or changing institutional protocols as a means of correcting problems identified by QI programmes are given below in the section "Closing the loop".

Targeted education

Educational opportunities include existing methods such as daily ward rounds, departmental grand rounds, regularly scheduled conferences, and case presentations. Other less routine but excellent educational opportunities include periodic journal clubs to highlight and openly discuss influential and controversial publications, as well as focused reading groups on specific topics of interest. Alternative educational options include newsletters, posters and videos from professional societies and health ministries. Many of these types of educational materials do not require the physical presence of a practitioner in a scheduled meeting and therefore can be accessed by the clinician when convenient.

A typical example of a targeted educational effort that might be identified by the QI process follows. By evaluating recent trauma deaths, the QI process may reveal that a problem exists with regard to patients with pelvic fractures. A number of patient deaths secondary to pelvic fractures and associated pelvic haemorrhage might be discovered as part of the QI technique of preventable death panel reviews. So if the QI process has now identified a problem, what is a possible corrective strategy to fix this problem? A method that potentially decreases mortality secondary to haemorrhage from pelvic fracture is early external reduction and stabilization of the fracture in the emergency department. A simple, easily available and cost-effective method for initial pelvic stabilization is pelvic "binding" or "sheeting". Although, the concept of pelvic sheeting is relatively simple and cheap, the actual specifics of where and how to apply the binding sheet effectively can best be relayed to clinicians through a targeted teaching session. The targeted educational session should include direct hands-on practice of the technical aspects of how to apply pelvic binding in patients with a pelvic fracture. Additionally, an essential component of this type of targeted educational experience is a thorough discussion, which should include a question-and-answer component on the indications, and explanation of the small tricks that make application of the binding sheet more effective in optimally reducing fracture, the length of the binding, and the advantages and disadvantages of using the technique of sheeting in patients with pelvic fractures.

It is often useful to hold joint educational conferences with other services that are closely involved in caring for trauma patients. Regularly scheduled combined teaching conferences can discuss evidence-based guidelines, difficult cases, and other relevant topics. Such teaching conferences can involve two or more services such as general surgery, emergency medicine, anaesthesiology, orthopaedics, neurosurgery, and others. These conferences can be a valuable means of disseminating knowledge and can serve as a platform for establishing friendly relationships while not in the stressful circumstances that often surround a critically injured patient.

These conferences are both an essential part of the learning process and a forum for providing feedback on outcomes, both good and bad, to practitioners who had an important responsibility for patient care at a particular point in time but who do not continue to care for a patient throughout the course of hospitalization. Providing positive feedback on patient outcomes within a non-stressed environment also builds positive relationships when a particular practitioner's contribution to the care of the patient is publicly acknowledged and appreciation is expressed. Openly acknowledging successes in an educational context also makes frank discussions about poor outcomes more likely to be constructive.

Some trauma centres find that holding periodic journal clubs in conjunction with other specialties at a location away from the hospital provides a very friendly and non-threatening opportunity for clinicians to interact without the constant clinical demands of the hospital setting. Even if held infrequently – perhaps quarterly or twice a year – these educational opportunities can have a significant and durable positive impact by improving communication, interaction between clinicians and, ultimately, quality of care.

Actions for improvement targeted at specific providers

Although most corrective strategies identified in the QI process address systems issues, there are occasions when the actions of a specific provider must be addressed. This may be either because of a particularly problematic issue or because of a pattern of unacceptable performance. This area is a relatively small component of QI, and it is important to emphasize that, as far as possible, corrective strategies aimed at specific practitioners should be constructive. As emphasized in the 12 basic elements of QI (Table 3), educational evaluations and provider improvement interventions must be critical but not destructive. Respect for the opinions and role of the deliverers of health care is essential. Accusatory methods must be avoided. Peer review processes and targeted interventions must be uniform, non-political and honest, and should incorporate evidence-based medicine. The three potential corrective strategies focusing on individual providers include counselling, further training and, when all else fails, a change in privileges or credentials.

Counselling: Counselling can be relevant for doctors, nurses and other staff when behavioural issues pose a problem. Counselling can be performed by the chief of the hospital or by the head of a department for doctors, or by a nurse manager for nursing staff. Counselling should occur in a timely fashion after any incident that merits intervention. Discussions are best held in private, or in small groups if more than one individual is involved. Counselling can be very difficult, but at times it is necessary. Discussions should be documented and followed up. Bearing in mind standard behavioural theory, any positive responses or reactions as a result of counselling should be acknowledged and rewarded in order to optimize the effectiveness of the process and to reinforce positive behaviour patterns.

Further training: At times, further training is a useful corrective strategy. If technical issues in clinical care arise, providers can be referred to highly specific and intensive courses that emphasize clinical management. Examples of such courses are included in section 5. Alternatively, further training may be behaviour improvement, such as training in conflict resolution training for staff who exhibit negative interactions under stressful conditions.

Changes in privileges or dismissal from practice: When efforts to effect positive change in a particular provider through counselling or further training are not successful, on rare occasions a change in privileges or possibly dismissal from practice at the hospital must be undertaken. Such extremes are unusual corrective strategies and require implementation at high levels within the hospital (such as the medical staff office as well as the department head). Restriction of privileges or dismissal from patient care should be reserved for occasions when other corrective action plans have failed. The potential for dismissal from practice at an institution or for restricting or denying privileges underscores the need for integrating trauma QI with hospital QI processes. The potential for dismissal also emphasizes the importance of documenting any prior corrective strategies and efforts implemented to improve performance in order to avoid controversy.

Enhanced resources, facilities, or communication

On occasion, a critical shortage or deficiency in resources repeatedly interferes with the process of caring for a patient. Rectifying the deficiency may be achieved by improved organization and planning without the need for high-cost solutions. One example is to make sure that resources that are necessary in emergency situations are readily accessible. This may in turn imply activities such as making sure that chest tube stocks are checked daily in order to ensure adequate availability when urgently needed, developing a "difficult airway cart" with multiple advanced options for obtaining an emergency airway, or designing a designated "surgical airway tray" that is always available should other means of securing an airway fail.

Communication issues can often be resolved with simple solutions. Making sure that all staff wear their name badges correctly and that the print is large enough to be easily readable from across a room can improve communication in an active chaotic trauma resuscitation area or casualty ward. To make a blood bank aware of an acute situation requiring immediate availability of blood products, one can create a "massive transfusion protocol" as was discussed in the section on guidelines, pathways and protocols. Then, just stating the words "activate the massive transfusion protocol" sends a clear message to the staff manning the blood bank of the emergent nature of the situation so they may prioritize their work efforts.

Delays in communication can often be solved by having designated cell phones for staff on call. Access to the operating room for emergencies can be improved by providing direct cell phones to be carried by the on-call operating theatre charge nurse and anaesthesiologist (Performance Improvement Subcommittee of the American College of Surgeons Committee on Trauma, 2002). The example of the QI programme in Khon Kaen, Thailand, demonstrated that delays in care of the injured could be improved by a network of radios within the hospital.

The above are brief examples that address local circumstances. Defining appropriate, affordable and sustainable resource enhancement in any given circumstance depends on having a QI process that can provide meaningful data on the problems that should be the targets of corrective action.

Closing the loop

A very important component of QI is "loop closure". QI must demonstrate that corrective actions have had the intended effect. Closing the loop implies that the process or outcome has been measured after implementation of the corrective strategy, and that improvement has been demonstrated. Some loops may never be completely closed, but may require ongoing monitoring and efforts to continually improve problems (Performance Improvement Subcommittee of the American College of Surgeons Committee on Trauma, 2002; American College of Surgeons, 2006). There follow several examples of both situations of loop closure.

A QI programme in the United States had noted an unacceptable frequency of deaths from errors of under-appreciation of intra-thoracic haemorrhage due to clotting of a chest tube. A protocol was developed to address this by mandating placement of a second chest tube in all patients whose initial chest tube drained more than 10 ml/kg of blood. Likewise, when this occurred, the protocol mandated that the attending (consultant) surgeon should be notified of this case as a high priority for surgery. As indicated in Table 19, this simple protocol change virtually eliminated the problem, as demonstrated by continued monitoring by the trauma QI programme. In similar fashion, this same programme identified several deaths that had occurred because unstable patients were transferred from other hospitals and arrived with inadequate

TABLE 19 **Examples of loop closure for two corrective actions targeted towards problems identified in a trauma QI programme**

Error group	1996	1997	1998	1999	2000	2001	2002	2003	2004
Uncontrolled thoracic haemorrhage	●	●●●	●			●			
Interhospital transfer of unstable patient	●●								

Table shows deaths per year associated with particular errors, before (white) versus after (grey) institution of corrective measures.
Source: Gruen et al., (2006). Reproduced by permission of the Annals of Surgery.

notice and preparation. Institution of a process for better receiving phone calls from transferring hospitals resulted in better communication among hospital staff as to preparations necessary for transferred patients (Gruen et al., 2006).

An example of a loop closure that might require continuous monitoring is the institution of a massive transfusion protocol. A trauma QI process might identify an "area for improvement" in timely access and administration of blood products in severely haemorrhaging patients. If a hospital or region has a blood bank available, a standardized communication process for obtaining blood products might be instituted as a corrective strategy. The creation or updating of the communication protocol with the blood bank would be an example of loop closure. However, this type of loop closure would require ongoing monitoring every time the protocol was activated to ensure that the process for obtaining blood products in a timely fashion continued to meet the needs of the patient and practitioners (Malone, Hess and Fingerhut, 2006; Gonzalez et al., 2007).

4.6 System-wide and prehospital quality improvement

Most of the above techniques have focused on QI for hospital-based trauma care. However, it is important to emphasize that QI can be used to strengthen trauma care more broadly, including in the prehospital setting and in region-wide trauma care systems that encompass prehospital care and networks of hospitals. Likewise, QI for acute care should complement or, ideally, be integrated with QI for rehabilitation (American College of Surgeons, 2006; Hoyt, Coimbra and Potenza, 2008).

Some of the best examples of the usefulness of QI techniques to identify problems and direct and stimulate corrective action come from region-wide trauma care systems. As just one example, a preventable death review in California, USA, in the 1970s showed a high rate of preventable deaths in Orange County. One third of the deaths due to head injuries and two thirds of the deaths due to injuries elsewhere in the body were judged preventable. This was in comparison to very few such preventable deaths in the neighbouring San Francisco County. This review stimulated corrective action in the form of better organization of trauma care services in Orange County, including designation of and investment in several main hospitals for trauma care and the enactment of prehospital triage criteria to bring the most severely injured to these hospitals. The result was a notable decrease in medically preventable deaths (West and Trunkey, 1979; West, Cales and Gazzaniga, 1983).

Many of the prior techniques explained in this book are amenable to use in both facility-based and prehospital settings. However, as many of the examples and experiences that have been provided are from hospital settings, we now review several considerations specific to prehospital trauma care. These are oriented for the circumstances in which there is an existing ambulance service (e.g. formal emergency medical services or EMS).

Prehospital trauma QI is made somewhat more difficult by the lack of an evidence base for several of the procedures used, such as IV fluids and advanced airway management (e.g. endotracheal intubation). Although these are definitely well established techniques for the care of the injured in general, their effectiveness in the prehospital setting has not been well defined (Bickell et al., 1994; Bunn et al., 2001; Maier and Rhodes, 2001; Sasser et al., 2005). Nonetheless, several well-accepted measures of quality are often monitored in the prehospital setting (Soreide and Grande, 2001; Hoyt, Coimbra and Potenza, 2008), namely:

- timeliness of arrival and of transport;
- dispatch of appropriate personnel (i.e. personnel with training and skills appropriate for the level of acuity of the emergency to which they are responding, in systems in which there are different levels of providers to choose from);
- airway management, including success of endotracheal intubations (in systems in which that technique is utilized in the prehospital setting);
- spinal immobilization;
- outcome, including evaluation of the contribution of the prehospital component of care to preventable deaths.

There are also several considerations for implementation of QI specific to the prehospital setting. From the viewpoint of the supervisor (whether medical director or otherwise) of an EMS system, it is useful regularly to review the documents written by prehospital care providers (e.g. EMS runsheets). In general, poor documentation is often indicative of poor quality care (Sasser et al., 2005).

In the review of the records, it is especially useful to identify and follow-up on "critical incidents". These include obvious mistakes, unexpected poor outcome, and near misses (for more details on these concepts, see section 4.3). Review of these critical incidents with prehospital personnel is similar to the M & M reviews in-hospital. The review seeks to identify root causes, conditions, and policies that may have contributed to the problem (Sasser et al., 2005).

It is also useful to undertake periodic reviews of common conditions, such as motor vehicle crashes, to assess their outcomes, such as by obtaining follow-up from the hospital. These reviews combine such outcome data with the EMS data on process of care, thus giving medical directors a quantitative overview of the functioning of the system (Sasser et al., 2005).

The above methods can be supplemented by regular listening-in on the radio (when technically feasible) and by direct field observation of the performance of prehospital providers.

When problems are identified, a variety of corrective actions can be instituted, namely:

- periodic retraining in the basics of prehospital care;
- educational sessions in which new procedures or techniques are introduced or existing ones modified;
- educational sessions in which staff are oriented to new equipment or medications;
- giving feedback from the auditing of radio communication, direct observation, and review of case reports;
- discipline (Clarifying expectations or providing supplemental training will usually correct identified problems, whether by individuals or system-wide. However, for the few cases where this is not the case, the EMS supervisor must have the authority to maintain discipline and suspend or dismiss prehospital providers who consistently do not meet expectations) (Sasser et al., 2005).

The above prehospital QI techniques apply whether one considers a specific EMS service (e.g. one ambulance service) or all EMS services in a given area or network. They can also be applied as part of a hospital QI programme which monitors prehospital care as part of the spectrum of care for cases received at that facility, with feedback provided as appropriate to the EMS services that transported the patients.

Finally, QI processes, whether for hospitals or broader systems, often have legal connotations. In most legal systems, QI processes and the minutes/records that they generate are considered confidential and legally protected. That is, they cannot be released publicly and they are not legally "discoverable" or subject to release by subpoena by outside parties. They are thus regarded in a similar light to discussions held between individuals and their lawyers or their clergy. This is to maintain frankness and openness in the reporting of errors and problems by the QI participants. When new QI programmes are being set up in locations where they have not previously existed, it would be useful to ensure the confidentiality of the discussions and related minutes/records and accord legal protection to them.

4.7 Role of medical records and trauma registry

There is a need for adequate data to support the QI process, no matter what type of QI activity is undertaken. For M & M conferences these data are often readily available even from the most basic of medical records systems. As M & M conferences are usually conducted within a few days or weeks of the event, the recorded information can be augmented by discussions with the care providers who were directly involved with the cases in question. For preventable death panel reviews, there is a need for somewhat more functional medical records systems, as most reviews are retrospective. In many locations, both of the above methods have been held back by lack of adequate documentation (Mock, 2007). This is often the result of minimal recording of information at the time of service provision, especially for cases which expire soon after arrival at the hospital, cases on which the QI process should specifically focus (London et al., 2001). Thus, a component of instituting or improving QI activities may involve improving the adequacy of documentation of trauma care in the medical records, especially in the early phases of care. Such improved documentation would be both for day-to-day management and for aiding QI monitoring and management of care in the longer term. Any such efforts to improve record-keeping need to be seen as beneficial by care providers and should therefore not be unduly cumbersome or time consuming (Kobusingye and Lett, 2000).

More advanced QI methods, such as tracking of audit filters and complications and especially statistical methods, require more advanced medical records (health information) systems. In many cases, this implies a trauma registry. A trauma registry is built upon, but is distinct from, the more general medical records system. A trauma registry may be defined as "a disease-specific collection composed of a file of uniform data elements that describe the injury event, demographics, prehospital information, diagnosis, care, outcomes, and costs of treatment for injured patients" (American College of Surgeons, 2006). In most cases it is computerized, permitting ease of analysis and tracking of QI data elements. It is this ease of analysis and ability to track specific data (such as complications or process-of-care measures), as well as ability to adjust for severity of injury, that distinguish trauma registries from general medical records systems.

An in-depth review of trauma registries is beyond the scope of this publication. For more details, readers are referred to several publications on this topic (Holder et al., 2001; Mock, 2001; American College of Surgeons, 2006; Nwomeh et al., 2006). Some pertinent features of trauma registries are described below, as they pertain to QI activities.

Trauma registries differ at different facilities as to inclusion and exclusion criteria, data elements collected, and software used. Most use a fairly standard inclusion criteria as to diagnoses, including data on most patients with ICD codes ranging from 800.00 to 959.9. Depending on the specific registry, a level of severity is often used, with patients being included in the registry if they are admitted to the hospital at all, admitted for more than 24 hours, or admitted for more than three days. Generally, any trauma death at the facility is also included. Some registries exclude specific ICD codes, such as those representing late effects of injury, isolated hip fractures, or foreign body aspiration (American College of Surgeons, 2006; Nwomeh et al., 2006).

Data recorded in registries include several variables from each of the following categories: demographics, mechanism of injury and related location and circumstances, prehospital information, vital signs (both prehospital and at emergency department arrival), diagnoses (e.g. ICD[3] codes), level of severity of injury (whether by GCS, ISS, RTS, TRISS or another score), procedures performed (including operations), outcome (including length of stay), complications, and data on costs and resource utilization. The American College of Surgeon's National Trauma Data Bank collects data on 76 variables. Many hospital-based trauma registries collect data on more (American College of Surgeons, 2006; Nwomeh et al., 2006).

Various proprietary registry software packages are available. Many can be run either on stand-alone PCs or on hospital networks. However, it is important to note that many successful registries have been created using low-cost (or even free), simple-to-use software such as Epi-Info (Centers for Disease Control and Prevention, 2008).

There is a growing experience with trauma registries in low-income and middle-income countries. In Uganda, Kobusingye and Lett (2000) reported on the establishment of a 19-item registry, which permitted severity adjustment using the locally developed Kampala Trauma Score. This registry was created using the freely available programme Epi-Info. In Pakistan, a more extensive registry was established which utilized severity adjustment with TRISS. This has proved very useful for identification of problems to target in the local QI process (Zafar et al., 2002; Jat et al., 2004). The previously noted example of the QI programme in Khon Kaen, Thailand, relied extensively on the trauma registry created at that institution. In Zaria, Nigeria, Nwomeh et al. (2006) reported on the institution of a registry for injured children, which derived data from a single-sheet, 10-item form. It is notable that, due to resource restrictions, this has been maintained in paper format (not computerized). Nonetheless, it has been useful for identifying issues that were then targeted to improve care of injured children and has resulted in reorganization of paediatric trauma care at their facility (Nwomeh et al., 2006).

Thus, in many circumstances QI efforts need to address improvements in data collection and use. This can imply better recording of data at the time of patient presentation. It can imply better handling and availability of that data from standard medical record systems. In some circumstances, it can imply

---

[3] The *International classification of diseases and related health problems* (ICD), published by WHO, is currently in its 10th revision.

establishment of a formal trauma registry, which can be done in an affordable, sustainable and simple fashion.

4.8 Appropriateness of different techniques at different levels of the health care system

The recommendations contained in this book can be implemented at any level of the health care system. The most optimal QI techniques depend on the level of the health care system, the trauma volume of the facility, and the current status of trauma QI activities.

For tertiary care centres or other large hospitals with multiple specialties and high trauma volumes, all techniques described in this book are potentially relevant, depending on the existing status of QI activities. If absolutely no QI activities are in use, starting basic M & M conferences would be the basic step. If, as is the case in most larger hospitals in low-income and middle-income countries, M & M conferences are in regular use, two further steps can be considered.

The first is to derive more benefit from the existing conferences by way of improving the methodology of how they are conducted – and especially by increasing the rigour with which problems are identified and corrective action is suggested and followed up – and by instituting the concept of "closing the loop". Similarly, the M & M conferences can be augmented by additional, periodic multi-departmental reviews of cases selected from the departmental M & Ms and by review of summary statistics from the individual departmental M & M conferences.

The second step is to institute more formal review of expired cases through preventable death panel reviews. This could be a component of the multi-department reviews. Such panel reviews typically help to engage stakeholders from several different departments. They also provide a more standardized way to define preventability and to identify problems. They can create consensus on corrective action, which will help with the creation of political will to institute such action. For preventable death reviews, a very useful additional piece of information is the autopsy. Given cultural restrictions concerning autopsy in some locations, it must be emphasized that much can be done without autopsy data. However, when available, autopsy reports do provide useful clues for the work of preventable death panels. Moreover, autopsies are already being conducted in many locations for many trauma deaths for forensic reasons. Autopsy rates for trauma deaths are well above 50% for many larger hospitals in Africa, Asia and Latin America (Mock, 2007). As autopsy reports with more accurate information on anatomical cause of death are so readily available, it would make sense to use this important information in preventable death reviews and other QI activities.

If the above methods are already in use, further steps to be considered would include tracking of audit filters and complications and use of statistical means for severity adjustment. These methods offer more objectivity in identifying problems and better means for tracking the results of corrective action. The previously reported programmes from Thailand and Pakistan indicate the potential utility of these methods in hospitals in developing countries (Chardbunchachai, Suppachutikul and Santikarn, 2002; Jat et al., 2004). These methods depend on the existence of a well-organized source of regular data, which in most cases would imply the creation of a trauma registry.

The above considerations can be applied to QI in general, with trauma cases being a component of the cases reviewed. However, for hospitals with especially high trauma volumes (such as above 1000 or 2000 trauma admissions per year), a specific trauma QI programme might be warranted, given the specific nature of problems to be identified and corrective action to institute.

For medium-sized hospitals that have a smaller range of specialties, many of the above considerations can still apply, especially if they are very busy with trauma. However, if not, considerable benefit can still accrue from making sure that trauma cases are well addressed in general basic QI activities such as M & M conferences. The same sequence of progression to preventable panel reviews, tracking of audit filters and complications, and statistical risk adjustment methods pertains, depending on trauma volume, local priorities, and resource availability.

For smaller hospitals (such as hospitals staffed primarily by general practitioners) and networks of clinics, addressing trauma QI may still be important, especially for those facilities that receive considerable numbers of trauma cases, such as those along major roads. However, it is unlikely that a dedicated QI programme focusing specifically on trauma would be warranted. Broader management information systems that address both efficiency and quality improvement of a broad range of issues are likely to be required (WHO, 1998).

Moreover, it is to be noted that networks of clinics, smaller hospitals, and medium-sized hospitals often play a substantial role in region-wide trauma care, as they are often the first level of referral to higher facilities. In some cases their role interacts and overlaps with prehospital care in the area. Thus, region-wide efforts to improve trauma care and better establish trauma systems need to consider this "base of the pyramid" of trauma care. Likewise, region-wide trauma QI activities will of necessity incorporate cases handled at these facilities. In more advanced systems, this can be done through the establishment of region-wide trauma registries and more formal region-wide trauma QI work. More generally however, region-wide preventable death panel reviews could serve as a means to identify problems in the process of trauma care at smaller facilities. Moreover, constructing the panels to include care providers from these facilities will help to create political will to institute the necessary corrective action.

The specifics of which QI techniques might be utilized at what level of the health care system or in region-wide activities will vary with many local considerations. However, there is almost certainly a role for better monitoring of the process of trauma care through some type of QI activity at any level of the health care system and in any location where there are significant numbers of trauma patients.

When deciding how to start completely new QI activities or to expand on existing ones, two basic principles apply at all levels of the health care system. The first is to be realistic and to build up slowly and sustainably. Taking small initial steps and addressing the main priorities (such as obviously preventable deaths) will lay the ground work for longer-term successes. For example, as discussed above, a hospital with ongoing but relatively ineffective M & M conferences might best start by improving the procedural rigour with which the conferences are conducted and by better identifying and following up on corrective strategies.

The second basic principle is to engage with and gain the cooperation of a range of stakeholders, including hospital administration, clinicians from several different specialities and, in the case of system-wide QI, prehospital providers and governmental authorities responsible for the area's network of health care institutions. Any QI activities must have adequate mandate to gather the needed information and to implement the corrective action plan that is agreed on. Broad political support is equally necessary to assure that such corrective action is successful.

5. Overlap of these guidelines with other activities

5.1 Clinical algorithms

This publication presents guidance on the implementation of QI programmes. These programmes will also be based on the participants' knowledge of and expertise in the specifics of clinical trauma care and local standards of best practice. The QI process seeks to make sure that local standards are met. The current publication does not deal with such specific clinical issues. What standards, clinical guidelines or algorithms exist, are in place locally, or should be in place locally needs to be determined by clinicians and administrators in each location. There are, however, several resources that provide guidance as to what would constitute good trauma care, and participants in the QI process may utilize these as needed. These include textbooks of surgery and of trauma care which are considered authoritative, many of which are published in individual countries and are written with local conditions in mind.

For initial management, including initial resuscitation and diagnostic work-up, several courses have been developed which lay out well developed protocols for care. These include, among others, Advanced Trauma Life Support, or ATLS (American College of Surgeons, 2008), National Trauma Management Course, or NTMC (Academy of Traumatology, 2009), Primary Trauma Care, or PTC (Wilkinson and Skinner, 2000), and Trauma Nursing Core Course, or TNCC (Emergency Nurses Association, 2009). For standards for prehospital care, similar courses with related protocols include International Trauma Life Support, or ITLS (Campbell, 2007), and PreHospital Trauma Life Support, or PHTLS (National Association of Emergency Medical Technicians, 2006). Going beyond the initial management, Definitive Surgical Trauma Care (DSTC) lays out protocols for operative management.

There are also several sets of guidelines that may be used in the development of individual institutional protocols. These may be found on the following web sites: http://www.east.org
http://www.learnicu.org/Quick_Links/Pages/default.aspx

Several particularly useful references for clinical trauma care in the setting of smaller (first-referral level) hospitals in low-income and middle-income countries have been developed by WHO's Department of Essential Health Technology. These are particularly oriented to circumstances where resources are limited and where general doctors need to undertake basic operative care (of trauma and other conditions) without access to specialists and often with limited capabilities for urgent referral. These references include the textbook *Surgical care at the district hospital* and educational materials from the *Integrated management for emergency and essential surgical care (IMEESC) tool kit* (WHO, 2003; WHO, 2007). Both are freely available on the WHO web site.

The above lists of references are meant to give general guidance on resources for information on clinical best practices for trauma care. The lists are not meant to be all-encompassing and there are other references that are useful for QI programmes.

5.2 Patient safety

There is a growing worldwide movement towards assuring greater patient safety in health care. WHO has its own Patient Safety Programme which is part of the World Alliance for Patient Safety. During the past few years, the Alliance has worked on several efforts including the "Global Patient Safety Challenges". The first is on preventing health-care associated infections by promoting better hand hygiene among health care workers. The second challenge is "Safe Surgery Saves Lives". The WHO programme promotes the use of a standardized surgical safety checklist for all operating rooms to ensure that nothing is forgotten in the complex peri-operative patient care process, from pre-operative preparation to post-operative management. It is especially oriented to preventing errors such as wrong site surgery and anaesthetic complications. It is also intended to improve communication between members of the operating team. This one-page checklist has been pilot-tested in eight hospitals, including at least one on each continent, and in low-income, middle-income and high-income countries. It has met with considerable interest and acceptance by surgical organizations globally and has been shown to lower peri-operative complications and mortality (Humphreys, 2008; Haynes et al, 2009). The efforts of the "Safe Surgery Saves Lives" challenge fits closely with the goals of trauma QI, in that safe operations are a major component of what trauma QI seeks to assure.

In similar manner, the Joint Commission International (JCI) has been designated as a WHO Collaborating Centre on Patient Safety and works closely with the World Alliance for Patient Safety. It has been disseminating "patient safety solutions" that include ways to prevent common medication errors, to improve communication during patient handovers, and to avoid wrong site surgery (http://www.jcipatientsafety.org/29083/).

There are several other synergies between efforts to promote greater patient safety and efforts to promote greater implementation of trauma QI (WHO, 2006). These include:

- Both patient safety efforts and trauma QI promote the improvement of information systems in order to provide data to better understand and prevent errors. This fits precisely with the data needs of QI programmes, as discussed in section 4.7.
- The World Alliance for Patient Safety has especially noted the challenges of assuring safety in acute care, where risk of errors is increased by gaps in care caused by such issues as staffing constraints, shift work, and shortened time for processing data and decision-making. Trauma care is a significant component of such overall acute care.
- More than anything else, both efforts seek to change the organizational culture of health care institutions to promote greater emphasis on patient safety, and both seek to raise political commitment to patient safety.

Thus, people active in either field are strongly encouraged to join forces, especially at the local level, and promote changes that will assist each in achieving their mutual goals.

5.3 Strengthening of health care management

As noted previously, in many institutions QI for trauma cases will be handled as part of QI for the entire surgery department or even for an entire institution. Only larger institutions with high trauma volumes would be expected to have a specific programme for trauma QI.

Seen more broadly, QI for trauma care and for other clinical issues is a component of overall efforts to strengthen management of health services. WHO has a specific unit for this purpose, Organization and Management of Health Services (OMH), which is a team in the Department of Health System Governance and Service Delivery (HDS). This unit has developed a noteworthy set of resources and training materials for this purpose. These are freely available on their MAKER (Managers taking Action based on Knowledge and Effective use of Resources to achieve Results) web site (WHO, 2009).

The materials on the MAKER web site contain references and tools for strengthening health service management in general. There is an entire section on management of quality, including: quality assurance, standards, accreditation, user satisfaction, patient safety, and monitoring and evaluation of quality of care. Several in-depth references are provided for quality assurance in primary care. Although the latter are not directly related to QI for trauma care, there are definite synergies. Those seeking to promote greater use of trauma QI might find allies within similar movements in primary care and other fields.

References

Academy of Traumatology (2009). *National trauma management course.* Ahmedabad, Academy of Traumatology (India). (http://www.indiatrauma. org/, accessed 9 February 2009).

American College of Surgeons (2006). *Resources for optimal care of the injured patient.* Chicago, American College of Surgeons.

American College of Surgeons (2008). *Advanced trauma life support: student course manual, 8th edition.* Chicago, American College of Surgeons.

American College of Surgeons (2009). *National trauma data bank.* Chicago, American College of Surgeons. (http://www.facs.org/trauma/ntdb.html, accessed 9 February 2009).

Ammerman M (1998). *The root cause analysis handbook: a simplified approach to identifying, correcting, and reporting workplace errors.* New York, Quality Resources.

Association for the Advancement of Automotive Medicine (2005). *Abbreviated injury scale (AIS) 2005.* DesPlaines, IL, Association for the Advancement of Automotive Medicine.

Australian Commission on Safety and Quality in Health Care (2007). *Sentinel events in Australian public hospitals 2004–2005.* Canberra, Australian Institute of Health and Welfare.

Baker SP (1974). The injury severity score: a method for describing patients with multiple injuries and evaluating emergency care. *Journal of Trauma,* 14:187-196.

Bhatt R (1989). Professional responsibility in maternity care: role of medical audit. *International Journal of Gynaecology and Obstetrics,* 30:47-50.

Bickell WH et al. (1994). Immediate vs. delayed fluid resuscitation for hypotensive patients with penetrating torso injuries. *New England Journal of Medicine,* 331:1105-1109.

Boonmak P et al. (2005). Surveillance of anesthetic related complications at Srinagarind Hospital, Khon Kaen University, Thailand. *Journal of the Medical Association of Thailand,* 88(5):613-622.

Boyd CR, Tolson MA and CopesWS (1987). Evaluating trauma care: the TRISS method. Trauma Score and the Injury Severity Score. *Journal of Trauma,* 27(4):370-378.

Browne J et al. (2006). High quality acute care for the severely injured is not consistently available in England, Wales and Northern Ireland: report of a survey by the Trauma Committee, The Royal College of Surgeons of England.

Annals of the Royal College of Surgeons of England, 88(2):103-107.

Bunn F et al. (2001). *Effectiveness of prehospital care: a report by the Cochrane Injuries Group for the World Health Organization*. London, The Cochrane Injuries Group.

Campbell JE (2007). *International trauma life support, 6th edition*. Englewood Cliffs, NJ, Prentice-Hall.

Campbell WB (1988). Surgical morbidity and mortality meetings. *Annals of the Royal College of Surgeons of England*, 70(6):363-365.

Centers for Disease Control and Prevention (2008). *EpiInfo*. Atlanta, GA, Centers for Disease Control and Prevention.

Chadbunchachai W et al. (2003). Study on performance following key performance indicators for trauma care: Khon Kaen Hospital 2000. *Journal of the Medical Association of Thailand*, 86(1):1-7.

Chadbunchachai W et al. (2001). The comparative study for quality of trauma treatment before and after the revision of trauma audit filter, Khon Kaen hospital 1998. *Journal of the Medical Association of Thailand*, 84(6):782-790.

Chakraborty S, D'Souza SA and Northrup RS (2000). Improving private practitioner care of sick children: testing new approaches in rural Bihar. *Health Policy and Planning*, 15(4):400-407.

Champion HR (1989). A revision of the trauma score. *Journal of Trauma*, 29:623-629.

Champion HR et al. (1990). The Major Trauma Outcomes Study: establishing national norms for trauma care. *Journal of Trauma*, 30(11):1356-1365.

Champion HR, Sacco WJ and Copes WS (1995). Injury severity scoring again. *Journal of Trauma*, 38(1):94-95.

Chang A et al. (2005). The JCAHO patient safety event taxonomy: a standardized terminology and classification schema for near misses and adverse events. *International Journal for Quality in Health Care*, 17:95-105.

Chardbunchachai W, Suppachutikul A and Santikarn C (2002). *Development of service system for injury patients by utilizing data from the trauma registry*. Khon Kaen, Thailand, Office of Research and Textbook Project, Khon Kaen Hospital. (ISBN: 974-294-569-1)

Choy YC, Lee CY and Inbasegaran K (1999). Anaesthesia incident monitoring study in Hospital Kuala Lumpur – the second report. *Medical Journal of Malaysia*, 54(1):4-10.

Civetta JM, Hudson-Civetta J and Ball S (1996). Decreasing catheter-related infection and hospital costs by continuous quality improvement. *Critical Care Medicine*, 24(10):1660-1665.

Clarke DL et al. (2008). Applying modern error theory to the problem of missed injuries in trauma. *World Journal of Surgery*, 32(6):1176-1182.

Collin GR (1999). Decreasing catheter colonization through the use of an antiseptic-impregnated catheter: a continuous quality improvement project. *Chest*, 115(6):1632-1640.

Copes WS et al. (1995). American College of Surgeons audit filters: associations with patient outcome and resource utilization. *Journal of Trauma*, 38(3):432-438.

Cryer HG et al. (1996). Continuous use of standard process audit filters has limited value in an established trauma system. *Journal of Trauma*, 41(3):389-394; discussion 394-395.

DiRusso S et al. (2001). Preparation and achievement of American College of Surgeons level I trauma verification raises hospital performance and improves patient outcome. *Journal of Trauma*, 51(2):294-299; discussion 299-300.

Donabedian A (1996). The effectiveness of quality assurance. *International Journal for Quality in Health Care*, 8(4):401-407.

Dumont A et al. (2006). Facility-based maternal death reviews: effects on maternal mortality in a district hospital in Senegal. *Bulletin of the World Health Organization*, 84(3):218-224.

Edmonds M (2004). *Adverse events, iatrogenic injury and error in medicine*. Adelaide, The University of Adelaide. (http://www.informatics.adelaide.edu.au/topics/Safety/ME-AdverseEvents.html, accessed 9 February 2009).

Emergency Nurses Association (2009). *Trauma nursing core course*. (http://www.ena.org/catn_enpc_tncc/tncc/, accessed 9 February 2009).

Esposito TJ et al. (1999). Analysis of preventable pediatric trauma deaths and inappropriate trauma care in Montana. *Journal of Trauma*, 47:243-251.

Goel A, Kumar S and Bagga M (2004). Epidemiological and Trauma Injury and Severity Score (TRISS) analysis of trauma patients at a tertiary care centre in India. *National Medical Journal of India*, 17:186-189.

Gonzalez EA et al. Fresh frozen plasma should be given earlier to patients requiring massive transfusion. *Journal of Trauma*, 62(1):112-119.

Gruen RL et al. (2006). Patterns of errors contributing to trauma mortality: lessons learned from 2,594 deaths. *Annals of Surgery*, 244(3):371-380.

Haynes AB et al. (2009). A Surgical Safety Checklist to reduce morbidity and mortality in a global population. *New England Journal of Medicine*, 360: 491-499.

Holder Y et al. (2001). *Injury surveillance guidelines*. Geneva, World Health Organization, 2001.

Hoyt DB, Coimbra R and Potenza BM (2008). Trauma systems, triage, and transport. In: Feliciano DV, Mattox KL and Moore EE. *Trauma, 6th edition*. New York, NY, McGraw-Hill (pp 57-82.

Humphreys G (2008). Checklists save lives. *Bulletin of the World Health Organization*, 86(7):501-502.

Hutter MM et al. (2006). Identification of surgical complications and deaths: an assessment of the traditional surgical morbidity and mortality conference compared with the American College of Surgeons-National Surgical Quality Improvement Program. *Journal of the American College of Surgeons*, 203(5):618-624.

Ifenne D et al. (1997). Improving the quality of obstetric care at the teaching hospital, Zaria, Nigeria. *International Journal of Gynaecology and Obstetrics*, 59(1002):S37-S46.

Inbasegaran K, Kandasami P and Sivalingam N (1998). A 2-year audit of perioperative mortality in Malaysian hospitals. *Medical Journal of Malaysia*, 53(4):334-342.

Institute of Medicine (1999). *To err is human: building a safer health system*. Kohn L, Corrigan J, and Donaldson M, eds. Washington, DC, National Academy Press.

Institute of Medicine (2001a). *Crossing the quality chasm: a new health system for the 21st century*. Washington, DC, National Academy Press.

Institute of Medicine (2001b). *Preserving public trust: accreditation and human research participant protection programs*. Washington, DC, National Academy Press.

Ivatury R et al. (2008). Patient safety in trauma: maximal impact management errors at a Level I trauma center. *Journal of Trauma*, 64:265-272.

Jat A et al. (2004). Peer review audit of trauma deaths in a developing country. *Asian Journal of Surgery*, 27:58-64.

JCAHO (2005). *Root cause analysis in health care: tools and techniques*. Oakbrook Terrace, IL, Joint Commission on Accreditation of Healthcare Organizations.

JHPIEGO (2008). *Quality improvement and performance improvement: different means to the same end?* Baltimore, MD, Johns Hopkins Program for International Education in Gynecology and Obstetrics. (http://www.reproline.jhu.edu/English/6read/6pi/pi_qi/piqi1.htm accessed 9 February 2009).

Ko CY, Maggard M and Agustin M (2005). Quality in surgery: current issues for the future. *World Journal of Surgery*, 29(10):1204-1209.

Kobusingye OC and Lett RR (2000). Hospital based trauma registries in Uganda. *Journal of Trauma*, 48:498-502.

Laxminarayan R et al. (2006). Advancement of global health: key messages from the Disease Control Priorities Project. *Lancet*, 367(9517):1193-1208.

Lock D (1994). *Gower handbook of quality management*. New York, NY, Gower Publishing Company.

London JA et al. (2001). Priorities for improving hospital based trauma care in an African city. *Journal of Trauma*, 51:747-753.

MacKenzie EJ et al. (1992). Inter-rater reliability of preventable death judgments. The Preventable Death Study Group. *Journal of Trauma*, 33(2):292-302; discussion 302-303.

Madzimbamuto FD (2003). A hospital response to a soccer stadium stampede in Zimbabwe. *Emergency Medicine Journal*, 20(6):556-559.

Maher D (1996). Clinical audit in a developing country. *Tropical Medicine and International Health*, 1(4):409-413.

Maier RV and Rhodes M (2001). Trauma performance improvement. In: Rivara FP, Cummings P, Koepsell TD, Grossman DC and Maier RV, eds. *Injury control: a guide to research and program evaluation*. New York, NY, Cambridge University Press.

Malone DL, Hess JR and Fingerhut A (2006). Massive transfusion practices around the globe and a suggestion for a common massive transfusion protocol. *Journal of Trauma*, 60(6 Suppl):S91-S96.

Mathews JJ et al. (1997). A burn center cost-reduction program. *Journal of Burn Care and Rehabilitation*, 18(4):358-563; discussion 357.

Mbaruku G and Bergstrom S (1995). Reducing maternal mortality in Kigoma, Tanzania. *Health Policy and Planning*, 10:71-78.

Mitchell F, Thal E and Wolferth C (1994). American College of Surgeons Verification/Consultation Program: analysis of unsuccessful verification reviews. *Journal of Trauma*, 37:557-564.

Mitchell F, Thal E and Wolferth C (1995). Analysis of American College of Surgeons Trauma Consultation Program. *Archives of Surgery*, 130:578-584.

Mock C (2001). Case series and trauma registries. In: Rivara FP, Cummings P, Koepsell TD, Grossman DC and Maier RV, eds. *Injury control: a guide to research and program evaluation*. New York, NY, Cambridge University Press.

Mock C (2007). *Report to International Association for Trauma Surgery and Intensive Care on course in quality improvement for trauma care*. Seattle, WA, Harborview Injury Prevention and Research Center.

Mock C et al. (2004). *Guidelines for essential trauma care*. Geneva, World Health Organization.

Mock C et al. (2006). Evaluation of trauma care capabilities in four countries using the WHO-IATSIC guidelines for essential trauma care. *World Journal of Surgery*, 30:946-956.

Murlidhar V and Roy N (2004). Measuring trauma outcomes in India: an analysis based on TRISS methodology in a Mumbai university hospital. *Injury*, 35:386-390.

National Association of Emergency Medical Technicians (2006). *Prehospital trauma life support, 6th edition*. Edinburgh, Mosby.

Noorani N, Ahmed M and Esufali ST (1992). Implementation of surgical audit in Pakistan. *Annals of the Royal College of Surgeons of England*, 74(2 suppl):28-31.

Nwomeh BC et al. (2006). History and development of trauma registry: lessons from developed to developing countries. *World Journal of Emergency Surgery*,

1:32.

O'Keefe G and Jurkovich GJ (2001). Measurement of injury severity and co-morbidity. In: Rivara FP, Cummings P, Koepsell TD, Grossman DC and Maier RV, eds. *Injury control: a guide to research and program evaluation*. New York, NY, Cambridge University Press.

O'Leary MR (1995). *Clinical performance data: a guide to interpretation*. Oakbrook Terrace, IL, The Joint Commission on Health Care Accreditation (pp 65-96).

Oakley PA (1994). Setting and living up to national standards for the care of the injured. *Injury*, 25:595-604.

Pathak L et al. (2000). Process indicators for safe motherhood programmes: their application and implications as derived from hospital data in Nepal. *Tropical Medicine and International Health*, 5:882-890.

Peabody JW et al. (2006). Improving the quality of care in developing countries. In: Jamison DT et al., eds. *Disease control priorities in developing countries, 2nd edition*. Oxford and New York, Oxford University Press for the World Bank (pp 1293-1307).

Performance Improvement Subcommittee of the American College of Surgeons Committee on Trauma (2002). *Trauma performance improvement reference manual*. Chicago, IL, American College of Surgeons (http://www.facs.org/trauma/publications/manual.pdf accessed 9 February 2009)

Punjasawadwong Y et al. (2007). Multicentered study of model of anesthesia related adverse events in Thailand by incident report (the Thai Anesthesia Incident Monitoring Study): methodology. *Journal of the Medical Association of Thailand*, 90(11):2529-2537.

Reason J (1995). Understanding adverse events: human factors. *Quality in Health Care*, 4(2):80-89.

Ronsmans C (2001). How can we monitor progress towards improved maternal health goals? *Studies in Health Services Organization and Policy*, 17:317-342.

Rosengart MR, Nathens AB and Schiff MA (2007). The identification of criteria to evaluate prehospital trauma care using the Delphi technique. *Journal of Trauma*, 62(3):708-713.

Sanddal ND, Esposito TJ and Hansen JD (1995). *Conducting rural preventable trauma mortality studies: a comprehensive guide to the acquisition and review of relevant data in a rural environment*. Bozeman, MT, Critical Illness and Trauma Foundation Inc.

Sasser S et al. (2005). *Prehospital trauma care systems*. Geneva, World Health Organization.

Scarpelini S, de Andrade JI and Dinis Costa Passos A (2006). The TRISS method applied to the victims of traffic accidents attended at a tertiary level emergency hospital in a developing country. *Injury*, 37(1):72-77.

Shackford SR et al. (1987). Assuring quality in a trauma system – the medical audit committee: composition, cost, and results. *Journal of Trauma*, 27:866-875.

Siddiqui A, Zafar H and Bashir S (2004). An audit of head trauma care and mortality. *Journal of the College of Physicians and Surgeons of Pakistan*, 14:173-177.

Soreide E and Grande CM (2001). *Prehospital trauma care*. New York, NY, Marcel Dekker, Inc.

Spath PL (1997). *Investigating sentinel events. How to find and resolve root causes: a simplified approach to identifying, correcting, and reporting workplace errors*. Forest Grove, OR, Brown-Spath & Associates.

Teixeira PG et al. (2007). Preventable or potentially preventable mortality at a mature trauma center. *Journal of Trauma*, 63(6):1338-1346; discussion 1346-1347.

Thomas B et al. (1997). Ultrasound evaluation of blunt abdominal trauma: program implementation, initial experience, and learning curve. *Journal of Trauma*, 42(3):384-388; discussion 388-390.

Trunkey DD. (1999) Invited commentary: panel reviews of trauma mortality. *Journal of Trauma*, 47(3 Suppl):S44-S45.

West J (1981). An autopsy method for evaluating trauma care. *Journal of Trauma*, 21:32-34.

West J and Trunkey D (1979). Systems of trauma care: a study of two counties. *Archives of Surgery*, 114:455-460.

West JG, Cales RH and Gazzaniga AB (1983). Impact of regionalization. The Orange County experience. *Archives of Surgery*, 118(6):740-744.

Wilkinson DA and Skinner MW (2000). *Primary trauma care manual: a manual for trauma management in district and remote locations*. Oxford, Primary Trauma Care Foundation. (Available from: http://www.fsm.ac.fj/library/E-Books/PrimaryTraumaCareManual.pdf,accessed 9 February 2009).

Wilson PF, Dell LD and Anderson GF (1993). *Root cause analysis: a tool for total quality management*. Milwaukee, WI, ASQC Quality Press.

WHO (1998). *District health facilities: guidelines for development and operations*. Manila, World Health Organization Regional Office for the Western Pacific.

WHO (2007). *Integrated management of emergency and essential surgical care (IMEESC) tool kit*. Geneva, World Health Organization. (http://www.who.int/surgery/publications/imeesc/en/index.html, accessed 9 February 2009).

WHO (2003). *Surgical care at the district hospital*. Geneva, World Health Organization.

WHO ed. (2006). *World Alliance for Patient Safety Forward Programme 2006-2007*. Geneva, World Health Organization.

WHO (2009). *MAKER: Managers taking Action based on Knowledge and Effective use of resources to achieve Results*. Geneva, World Health Organization. (http://

www.who.int/management/en/, accessed 9 February 2009)

Zafar H et al. (2002). Registry based trauma outcome: perspective of a developing country. *Emergency Medicine Journal*, 19(5):391-394.

Zafarghandi M, Modaghegh M and Roudsari B (2003). Preventable trauma death in Tehran: an estimate of trauma care quality in teaching hospitals. *Journal of Trauma*, 55:459-465.

Zeitz PS et al. (1993). Quality assurance management methods applied to a local level primary health care system in rural Nigeria. *International Journal of Health Planning and Management*, 8:235-244.

Annex 1
Details of literature review of benefits of trauma quality improvement

As discussed in section 3 (Benefits of quality improvement programmes), in order to ascertain the evidence base supporting the recommendations contained in these guidelines we conducted a review of the published literature on the effectiveness of trauma QI programmes. A very brief summary of that review is reported in Section 3. A more detailed summary is reported below. A full review article with an in-depth discussion of the articles identified in the search is currently in press (Juillard et al., 2009).

Search methods

A PubMed search was done to identify relevant articles in peer-reviewed journals. The search terms used included: "trauma quality assurance", "trauma preventable deaths", "trauma performance improvement", and "trauma continuous quality improvement". Articles were included if they were primarily oriented to the care of injured patients or focused on health services that directly involved the care of trauma patients. Additionally, a QI method had to be used to identify correctable deficiencies in patient care, generate interventions to improve the weakness detected, and evaluate the implemented solution through measurable outcomes in order for an article to be included. Articles were not included in the review if they described only QI methodology without evaluating the efficacy of an intervention, if they did not include utilization of QI measures to identify the problem requiring intervention, or if they relied only on subjective evidence (e.g. expert opinion surveys).

Articles found

The PubMed search yielded a total of 7212 journal articles. The majority of articles retrieved by this search were excluded by review of their titles alone and subsequently 380 abstracts were read. After review of the articles for relevance to the defined inclusion criteria, a total of 36 articles were identified for use as a basis to evaluate the efficacy of QI methods in trauma care settings. Most (30) of the articles identified discussed QI for trauma patients in the hospital context, while four addressed system-wide QI programmes, and two involved the prehospital setting.

Studies were grouped according to the outcomes evaluated in each (Table A1). When a study included several outcomes, the highest impact outcome assessed was listed by using the following prioritization (in decreasing order): mortality, other patient outcome, and process. Outcomes such as preventable deaths, error-related deaths, and overall mortality were considered to fall under "mortality". "Other" patient outcome was defined primarily as morbidity (infection, pressure ulcers, and other complications), but also included patient satisfaction and cost. "Process" indicators included items such as timely application of appropriate procedures, improved documentation and data collection, and emergency department turnaround times. Thirteen studies evaluated changes in mortality associated with QI, while other patient outcomes were the main outcome assessed in 12 studies, and process indicators were the main outcome assessed in 11 studies.

Findings

Of the 36 articles reviewed, the vast majority (34) found improvements in mortality, other outcome, or process, while only two studies detected no difference after a QI programme or method was implemented (Table A1). No article reported a worsening of any outcome from a QI programme.

In nine articles, the results of an overall QI programme were evaluated. Many of the articles reviewed demonstrated that comprehensive continuous quality improvement (CQI) programmes were associated with improvements in all three outcome categories (Yates et al., 1994; Gagneux, Lombrail and Vichard, 1998; DiRusso et al., 2001; Ruchholtz et al., 2001; Freeman et al., 2002; Welch and Allen, 2006). In one study, targeted QI measures in hip fracture patients resulted in a reduction of waiting time for operative procedure and pressure ulcers (Hommel, Ulander and Thorngren, 2003). In Thailand, use of audit filters and key performance indicators for trauma care QI was associated with a significant decrease in preventable deaths (Chadbunchachai et al., 2001; Chadbunchachai et al., 2003).

The QI implications of the introduction of trauma systems or dedicated hospital trauma teams were evaluated in six studies. City-wide and county-wide trauma services were found to result in a decrease of preventable deaths in Australia and California (Shackford et al., 1986; McDermott et al., 2007). Improved survival and decreased length of stay were associated with the introduction of a dedicated hospital-wide trauma team, while a dedicated paediatric trauma team was associated with a significant reduction of delayed diagnosis (Simons et al., 1999; Perno et al., 2005). In the United States, creation of a County Trauma Agency to coordinate trauma care among prehospital providers and state-designated trauma centres resulted in a decrease in preventable deaths from 23% to 7% (Thoburn et al., 1993). In a survey of 59 hospitals carried out in Quebec, the presence of a trauma performance improvement programme was found to be one of the factors most strongly correlated with improved outcomes (Liberman et al., 2005).

QI programmes specifically addressing prehospital care were the focus of two studies and were associated with decreased mortality and on-scene times, as well as improvements in chart documentation (O'Connor and Megargel, 1994; Eckstein and Alo, 1999).

Two studies found improvements in emergency department diagnostic tests. A QI team implemented changes intended to improve communication and consultation in order to reduce patient call-backs to the emergency department, which resulted in a 49% reduction in such call-backs (Preston et al., 1998). A pilot programme conducted by a QI team found that, when trauma surgeons were trained in abdominal ultrasound, they achieved 98% accuracy with a projected annual cost savings of US$100 000 (Thomas et al., 1997). However, one study showed no change in outcome. In this study, a QI programme which led to a change in procedures, in which radiologists specialized in abdominal imaging reviewed films read by board-certified or board-eligible radiologists generally did not lead to a change in patient outcomes or the process of care (Yoon et al., 2002).

Several articles evaluated the efficacy of QI programmes in reducing infections in intensive care units where trauma patients received care (Civetta, Hudson-Civetta and Ball, 1996; Collin, 1999; Cocanour et al., 2006). All these studies found that implementation of a QI process was associated with decreased rates of ventilator-associated pneumonia or catheter-related infections.

Many of the articles reviewed evaluated the implementation of forms and processes intended to improve documentation of patient care (Williams, Templeton and Smith, 1997; Nicol, 1999; Al Hussainy et al., 2004; Ritchie et al., 2004; Kanegaye et al., 2005; Ragoo and McNaughton, 2005). All these studies found an improvement in documentation related to QI programmes.

In several articles, the QI process was applied to specific problems identified in the care of injured patients (Aragon, 1999; Amato, Salter and Mion, 2006; Welch, 2006; Davidson, Griffin and Higgs, 2007). Results indicated an improvement in outcomes such as turnaround times in the emergency department, as well as a decrease in hypotension rates in patients with hip fractures, hypothermia rates in trauma patients, and restraint use in rehabilitation. One study involved a formal audit of all inpatient trauma deaths, and corresponding policy adjustments showed that changes in policy were associated with a decrease in error-related deaths (Gruen et al., 2006). A cost-reduction programme instituted in a burn centre resulted in decreased length of stay and infection rate, highlighting the parallel between cost-effectiveness and QI (Mathews et al., 1997). In only one of these studies was no improvement found. Treece et al (2004) implemented a "withdrawal of life support" order form in the intensive care unit setting, but found no change in the scores for comfort and quality in death and dying, nor for median time from ventilator withdrawal until death. However, physicians and nurses surveyed reported that they found the form helpful and total doses of comfort medications (narcotics and benzodiazepines) increased after the form was introduced.

Hence, this review has demonstrated that trauma QI programmes consistently improve the process of care, decrease mortality, and decrease costs. Further efforts to promote trauma QI globally are warranted.

TABLE A **Summary of literature review on effectiveness of trauma QI**

Article/type of QI Programme	Intervention	Outcome measure	Improvement
Comprehensive QI programme			
Chadbunchachai (2001)	Change in trauma audit filter using PAR	Preventable death rate	Y
Chadbunchachai (2003)	Implementation of KPIs in trauma care	Preventable death rate	Y
DiRusso (2001)	QI programme: ACS level I trauma verification	Mortality, length of stay, cost	Y
Freeman (2002)	QI programme: hip fracture patients	Pressure ulcers, pneumonia, wound infection	Y
Gagneux (1998)	QI programme: decrease adverse events	Adverse events	Y
Hommel (2003)	QI programme: hip fracture patients	Pressure ulcers, wait-time for operation	Y
Ruchholtz (2001)	QI programme: hospital-based trauma care	Mortality, process times	Y
Welch & Allen (2006)	QI programme: emergency-department based	Patient satisfaction, turnaround times	Y
Yates (1994)	QI programme: hospital-based trauma care	Adjusted mortality rate from severe injury	Y
Introduction of dedicated trauma services or systems			
Liberman (2005)	PI programme, prehospital notification	Decreased mortality	Y
McDermott (2007)	City-wide trauma system	Preventable deaths, scene time	Y
Perno (2005)	Dedicated paediatric trauma team	Delayed diagnosis	Y
Shackford (1986)	County-wide trauma system	Preventable deaths	Y
Simons (1999)	Dedicated hospital-wide trauma programme	Mortality, length of stay	Y
Thoburn (1993)	County-level coordination between prehospital providers and trauma centres	Mortality	Y

Prehospital care

Eckstein (1999)	QI programme to decrease scene times	Mortality, scene times	Y
O'Connor (1994)	QI programme to provide feedback to paramedics	ETI, charting, resuscitation, scene time	Y

Emergency department radiology

Preston (1998)	Team verifies radiographs read by ED physicians	Reduced callbacks	Y
Thomas (1997)	QI programme to evaluate trauma surgeon performance of abdominal ultrasound	Decreased diagnostic time, cost-saving	Y
Yoon (2002)	Verification of programme for ED radiology	Change in patient care due to QI read	N

Intensive care unit infection

Civetta (1996)	Catheter QI protocol	Catheter-associated infections	Y
Cocanour (2006)	"Ventilator bundle", auditing	Ventilator-associated pneumonia	Y
Collin (1999)	Evaluation and implementation of AICs	Catheter-associated infections	Y

Patient care documentation

Al Husainy (2004)	Proforma introduced for operative notes	Documentation of operative notes	Y
Kanegaye (2005)	Documentation form for pediatric wound care	Documentation of pediatric wound patients	Y
Nicol (1999)	Pre-printed form for sedation in ED	Documentation of consent/procedure details	Y
Ragoo & McNaughton (2005)	Proforma introduced for head injured patients	Documentation of head injured patients	Y
Ritchie (2004)	Pre-printed sticker: peri-operative antibiotics	Appropriate doses of antibiotics documented	Y
Williams (1997)	Trauma-specific patient charts	Improved documentation	Y
Treece (2004)	"Withdrawal of Life Support" order form	Time of ventilator withdrawal to death	N

QI method for specific problem

Amato (2006)	Comprehensive programme: decrease restraint use	Decreased restraint use, decreased fall rate	Y
Aragon (1999)	Multidisciplinary task force on hypothermia	Hypothermia	Y

Davidson (2007)	Protocol: fluid resuscitation in fracture patients	Hypotension	Y
Gruen (2006)	Review of preventable deaths, policy adjustments	Error-related deaths	Y
Mathews (1997)	Change in practice to decrease resource use	Decreased cost, infection	Y
Welch (2006)	DMADV implementation	Turnaround time in ED	Y

Abbreviations:
ACS: American College of Surgeons
AIC: Antibiotic impregnated catheters
CQI: Continuous quality improvement
DMADV: Define-Measure-Analyse-Devise-Verify methodology for root cause identification
ED: Emergency department
ETI: Endotracheal intubation (successful)
KPI: Key performance indicators
PAR: Participatory action research
PI: Performance improvement
QI: Quality improvement

References for Annex 1

Al Hussainy H et al. (2004). Improving the standard of operation notes in orthopaedic and trauma surgery: the value of a proforma. *Injury*, 35(11):1102-1106.

Amato S, Salter JP and Mion LC (2006). Physical restraint reduction in the acute rehabilitation setting: a quality improvement study. *Rehabilitation Nursing*, 31(6):235-241.

Aragon D (1999). Temperature management in trauma patients across the continuum of care: the TEMP Group. Temperature Evaluation and Management Project. *AACN Clinical Issues*, 10(1):113-123.

Chadbunchachai W et al. (2003). Study on performance following key performance indicators for trauma care: Khon Kaen Hospital 2000. *Journal of the Medical Association of Thailand*, 86(1):1-7.

Chadbunchachai W et al. (2001). The comparative study for quality of trauma treatment before and after the revision of trauma audit filter, Khon Kaen hospital 1998. *Journal of the Medical Association of Thailand*, 84(6):782-790.

Civetta JM, Hudson-Civetta J and Ball S (1996). Decreasing catheter-related infection and hospital costs by continuous quality improvement. *Critical Care Medicine*, 24(10):1660-1665.

Cocanour CS et al. (2006). Decreasing ventilator-associated pneumonia in a trauma ICU. *Journal of Trauma*, 61(1):122-129; discussion 129-130.

Collin GR (1999). Decreasing catheter colonization through the use of an antiseptic-impregnated catheter: a continuous quality improvement project. *Chest*, 115(6):1632-1640.

Davidson J, Griffin R and Higgs S (2007). Introducing a clinical pathway in fluid management. *Journal of Perioperative Practice*, 17(6):248-250, 255-256.

DiRusso S et al. (2001). Preparation and achievement of American College of Surgeons level I trauma verification raises hospital performance and improves patient outcome. *Journal of Trauma*, 51(2):294-299; discussion 299-300.

Eckstein M and Alo K (1999). The effect of a quality improvement program on paramedic on-scene times for patients with penetrating trauma. *Academic Emergency Medicine*, 6(3):191-195.

Freeman C et al. (2002). Quality improvement for patients with hip fracture: experience from a multi-site audit. *Quality and Safety in Health Care*, 11(3):239-245.

Gagneux E, Lombrail P and Vichard P (1998). Trauma emergency unit: long-term evaluation of a quality assurance programme. *Quality in Health Care*, 7(1):12-18.

Gruen RL et al. (2006). Patterns of errors contributing to trauma mortality: lessons learned from 2,594 deaths. *Annals of Surgery*, 244(3):371-380.

Hommel A, Ulander K and Thorngren KG (2003). Improvements in pain relief, handling time and pressure ulcers through internal audits of hip fracture patients. *Scandinavian Journal of Caring Sciences*, 17(1):78-83.

Juillard C et al. (2009). Establishing the evidence base for trauma quality improvement: a collaborative WHO-IATSIC review. *World Journal of Surgery*, March 17, Epub ahead of print.

Kanegaye JT et al. (2005). Improved documentation of wound care with a structured encounter form in the pediatric emergency department. *Ambulatory Pediatrics*, 5(4):253-257.

Liberman M et al. (2005). The association between trauma system and trauma center components and outcome in a mature regionalized trauma system. *Surgery*, 137(6):647-658.

Mathews JJ et al. (1997). A burn center cost-reduction program. *Journal of Burn Care and Rehabilitation*, 18(4):358-363; discussion 357.

McDermott FT et al. (2007). Management deficiencies and death preventability of road traffic fatalities before and after a new trauma care system in Victoria, Australia. *Journal of Trauma*, 63(2):331-338.

Nicol MF (1999). A risk management audit: are we complying with the national guidelines for sedation by non-anaesthetists? *Journal of Accident and Emergency Medicine*, 16(2):120-122.

O'Connor RE and Megargel RE (1994). The effect of a quality improvement feedback loop on paramedic skills, charting, and behavior. *Prehospital Disaster Medicine*, 9(1):35-38; discussion 38-39.

Perno JF et al. (2005). Significant reduction in delayed diagnosis of injury with implementation of a pediatric trauma service. *Pediatric Emergency Care*, 21(6):367-371.

Preston CA et al. (1998). Reduction of "callbacks" to the ED due to discrepancies in plain radiograph interpretation. *American Journal of Emergency Medicine*, 16(2):160-162.

Ragoo MA and McNaughton G (2005). Improving documentation of head injured patients admitted to the emergency department ward. *Scottish Medical Journal*, 50(3):99-100.

Ritchie S et al. (2004). Use of a preprinted sticker to improve the prescribing of prophylactic antibiotics for hip fracture surgery. *Quality and Safety in Health Care*, 13(5):384-387.

Ruchholtz S et al. (2001). [Interdisciplinary quality management in the treatment of severely injured patients. Validation of a QM system for the diagnostic and therapeutic process in early clinical management]. *Unfallchirurg*, 104(10):927-937.

Shackford SR et al. (1986). The effect of regionalization upon the quality of trauma care as assessed by concurrent audit before and after institution of a trauma system: a preliminary report. *Journal of Trauma*, 26(9):812-820.

Simons R et al. (1999). Impact on process of trauma care delivery 1 year after the introduction of a trauma program in a provincial trauma center. *Journal of Trauma*, 46:811-815.

Thoburn E et al. (1993). System care improves trauma outcome: patient care errors dominate reduced preventable death rate. *Journal of Emergency Medicine*, 11(2):135-139.

Thomas B et al. (1997). Ultrasound evaluation of blunt abdominal trauma: program implementation, initial experience, and learning curve. *Journal of Trauma*, 42(3):384-388; discussion 388-390.

Treece PD et al. (2004). Evaluation of a standardized order form for the withdrawal of life support in the intensive care unit. *Critical Care Medicine*, 32(5):1141-1148.

Welch S (2006). A wound-care process model improves emergency department turnaround time. *Journal for Healthcare Quality*, 28(3): 55-58.

Welch SJ and Allen TL (2006). Data-driven quality improvement in the emergency department at a level one trauma and tertiary care hospital. *Journal of Emergency Medicine*, 30(3):269-276.

Williams HR, Templeton PA and Smith RM (1997). An audit of trauma documentation. *Injury*, 28(3):165-167.

Yates DW et al. (1994). Trauma audit - closing the loop. *Injury*, 25(8):511-514.

Yoon LS et al. (2002). Evaluation of an emergency radiology quality assurance program at a level I trauma center: abdominal and pelvic CT studies. *Radiology*, 224(1):42-46.

Annex 2
Sample QI tracking form

As discussed in section 4.1 (Morbidity and mortality conferences), minutes should be taken during QI meetings to reflect the review, discussion, analysis, and proposed corrective action if applicable. Information may be better recorded by use of a standardized form. Such a form can help to make sure that important information is addressed in the peer review process, including discussion of corrective action. A sample of such a QI tracking form is included below.

Source: Figure 3 (Sample Performance Improvement Tracking Form), from Chapter 16 of American College of Surgeons (2006). *Resources for optimal care of the injured patient*. Chicago, American College of Surgeons. Reproduced by permission.

Figure 3. Sample Performance Improvement Tracking Form

Demographics	Source of Information (✓)	Location of Issue (✓)
Date of report _____	☐ Trauma nurse coordinator	☐ Prehospital
Medical record No._____	☐ Nurse management	☐ Resuscitation
Trauma registry No. _____	☐ Case manager	☐ Imaging
Attending No. _____	☐ PIPS coordinator	☐ Laboratory
Floor _____	☐ Patient relations	☐ Operating room
	☐ Risk management	☐ Postanesthesia care unit
	☐ Rounds	☐ Intensive care unit
	☐ Conference	☐ Floor
	☐ Registry	☐ Rehabilitation
	☐ Other	☐ Other

Complication, occurrence, problem, or complaint:

_____

_____

_____

_____

_____

Reported to _____ Reviewed by _____

Determination	Preventability	Corrective Action(s)	
☐ System-related	☐ Nonpreventable	☐ Unnecessary	☐ Peer review presentation
☐ Disease-related	☐ Potentially preventable	☐ Trend	☐ Resource enhancement
☐ Provider-related	☐ Preventable	☐ Education	☐ Process improvement team
☐ Cannot be determined	☐ Cannot be determined	☐ Guideline or protocol	☐ Privilege or credentialing action
		☐ Counseling	☐ Other _____

Comments:

_____

_____

_____

_____

Signature _____ Date_____

Annex 3
Sample data sheet for use in preventable death panel reviews

As discussed in section 4.2 (Preventable death panel review), the preparations for and conduct of panel reviews can be facilitated by using a standardized form. A sample case review form is included below. Part 1 is a data abstraction form to assist with gathering data from the medical record and other sources. Part 2 is a case review form to assist with recording the results of the panel's discussion, including decision on preventability of the death, identification of deficiencies in care, where the deficiencies occurred, and suggested corrective action.

Sample   **TRAUMA PREVENTABLE DEATH PANEL REVIEW**
         Page 1. Data Abstraction Form

Code number:

Age: Gender: M F

Mechanism of injury:

Time elapsed from injury to presentation to hospital (if known):

Time elapsed from presentation to hospital to death:

Site of death (circle one):

Prehospital   Casualty ward   ICU   Operating theatre   Ward   Other

Injuries sustained:

Injury Severity Score:

Abbreviated Injury Scale (AIS) by category:

Initial Systolic Blood Pressure:

Initial Glasgow Coma Scale score:

Description of course of treatment (if any):

Sample **TRAUMA PREVENTABLE DEATH PANEL REVIEW**
Page 2. Case Review Form Summarizing Decisions of Panel Review

Summary of panel discussion on preventability of the death:

....

....

....

....

....

Decision as to whether the death was:
   Definitely preventable
   Possibly preventable
   Not preventable
   Not preventable but treatment was suboptimal

Deficiencies in care (circle all that pertain):
   None
   Airway
   Haemorrhage
   Chest
   Fluid resuscitation
   Delays in treatment
   Other treatment problems
   Deficiencies in documentation

Location of deficiencies (if any, circle all that apply):
   Prehospital
   Casualty ward (emergency department)
   Operating theatre
   Intensive care unit
   Ward
   Interfacility transfer
   System inadequacy

Suggested corrective action:

....

....

....

....

Annex 4
Sample individual cases for review

As discussed in section 4.2 (Preventable death panel reviews), this annex contains summaries of cases to be used for practice for preventable death panel reviews and trauma QI reviews. These reinforce and provide examples of the principles discussed in the main part of this publication. The basic principles for the cases in this annex are based on cases that have been discussed at actual panel death reviews and QI programmes in several locations in different countries at different economic levels. Some reviews are for individual facilities and some for regional trauma systems. Details of demographics, injury-producing events, specific injuries, and specific aspects of care have been changed to protect the anonymity of the patients and providers. Any similarity to real people or cases in any location is purely coincidental.

Each case should be reviewed according to the following criteria:

1. Was this death or complication: definitely preventable; potentially preventable; not preventable; or not preventable, but care could have been improved?

2. What deficiencies in care occurred and where did they occur?
   - Possible deficiencies to consider include:
     - airway
     - haemorrhage control
     - chest
     - fluid resuscitation
     - delays in treatment
     - other
     - documentation.
   - Locations of deficiencies to consider include:
     - prehospital
     - emergency department (ED)
     - operating room (OR)
     - intensive care unit (ICU)
     - ward
     - interfacility transfer
     - system inadequacy.

3. What corrective actions should be taken?

These cases were reviewed by a QI committee in the area where they originated. Results of those discussions, along with further suggestions from the editors of this book, are provided after the case. The results of the prior QI committee reviews may or may not have been the best decisions on preventability and corrective action, but they represent the consensus of those who were involved in the QI activity locally and who were knowledgeable about the trauma systems in those areas. They provide a useful basis for further consideration by those using this publication. Readers should feel free to disagree with or to expand upon the recommendations from these prior discussions. Likewise, the main point of these cases is to gain experience in the use of QI methods. Specific points of clinical management may differ between locations and these cases are not meant to endorse specific clinical management algorithms. Finally, several cases discuss use of technology (e.g. various radiographic studies). These are based on what was available at the given location. Productive QI can be accomplished without any specific level of technology or resources and is equally likely to produce improvements in trauma care and its outcome in settings of high or low resource availability.

Acronyms used in case summaries:

BP	Blood Pressure
CE	Continuing Education
CPR	Cardio-Pulmonary Resuscitation
CT	Computerized Axial Tomography
CXR	Chest X-Ray
DC'd	Discontinued
DPL	Diagnostic Peritoneal Lavage
DVT	Deep Venous Thrombosis
ED	Emergency Department (also known in some locations as casualty ward)
FAST	Focused Assessment with Sonography in Trauma
GCS	Glasgow Coma Scale
GSW	Gun Shot Wound
ICU	Intensive Care Unit
M and M	Morbidity and Mortality Conferences
MVC	Motor Vehicle Crash
OR	Operating Room
ORIF	Open Reduction and Internal Fixation
PE	Pulmonary Embolus
QI	Quality Improvement
RBC	Red Blood Cell
SaO2	Arterial Saturation of Oxygen (usually as a reading from pulse oximetry)
SQ	Subcutaneous

Summary of cases in this annex

Section 1. Preventable death
1) Ruptured spleen, died while having X-rays
2) Head injury with respiratory distress
3) Death in ED from femoral artery laceration
4) Delayed presentation of head injury after a pedestrian injury
5) Retroperitoneal haematoma and orthopaedic injuries in a motorcyclist, death on ICU
6) Elderly female with multiple medical problems and prolonged time in OR for fixation of fractures

Section 2. Potentially preventable death
1) Multi-system organ failure after head and abdominal injury
2) Femur and pelvic fractures and facial lacerations
3) Death in ED from multiple injuries
4) Death in ICU after respiratory acidosis following drainage of subdural haematoma
5) Elderly man with bilateral traumatic above knee amputations
6) PE after chest injury

Section 3. Death not preventable, but care could be improved
1) Treatment in rural health centre before transfer for head injury
2) Extensive liver laceration
3) Liver laceration and colon injury in a motorcyclist; death in OR
4) Prolonged extrication, mesenteric avulsion, and cardiac arrest
5) Elderly male pedestrian in rural area

Section 4. Death not preventable
1) Death in OR with liver and spleen injuries
2) GSW to abdomen with cardiac arrest
3) PE after multiple orthopaedic injuries
4) Blunt cardiac injury and multiple abdominal injuries

Section 5. Non-fatal cases, but problems identified that required corrective actions
1) Infected impalement wound
2) Retained haemothorax

Section 1. **Preventable death**

1) Ruptured spleen, died while having X-rays

Case summary: 30-year-old male motorcyclist. He arrived at ED with a BP of 100/80 and a pulse of 120. He was slightly confused, with a GCS of 14. He was noted to have a deformity of his left thigh and an obvious open left tibia fracture, as well as injuries to his upper extremities. IV fluids were started and orthopaedic department was called. Requests for multiple extremity X-rays were made. Around 1 hour later, a repeat BP of 90/60 was recorded. Increased fluids were ordered. A little while later, he was taken to X-ray. After several of the X-rays were taken, the X-ray technician called the nurse to report that the patient looked very bad. He was found to be unconscious with a systolic BP of 40. Increased IV fluids were given. The doctor was called. By the time he arrived the patient had no vital signs. CPR started, but without success. Autopsy revealed mild cerebral oedema, a ruptured spleen with 4 litres of haemoperitoneum, left-sided orthopaedic injuries: humerus, radius and ulna, femur, and tibia (open).

Discussion: Patient died from ruptured spleen. There should have been more aggressive fluid resuscitation in the ED and a work-up for his abdominal status. With his decreased mental status, physical exam alone was not reliable. There was an over-emphasis on his orthopaedic injuries, with prolonged time waiting for and in X-ray. Deficiencies: haemorrhage control, fluids, and delays in treatment. Location of deficiency: ED.

Corrective actions:
- System improvement/enhanced resources: Improved staffing in ED, especially at peak times.
- Targeted education: Improved training for ED staff (doctors and nurses).
- Targeted education: Increased use of continuing education (CE), or in-service, courses for trauma care (as described in section 5.1), which were available but not fully utilized.
- Targeted education, provider counselling and communications training: Improved use of the concept of the "trauma team" with designated leader.
- Targeted education: Discussion session or grand rounds with topic being evaluation of abdominal trauma for blunt trauma.
- Targeted education: Training and review for providers in indications for use and the techniques of diagnostic peritoneal lavage and/or ultrasound to assess for haemoperitoneum.

- Systems improvement/enhanced resources: If an ultrasound machine is not already available, consideration of purchasing and/or stationing one in the ED to allow more rapid assessment for haemoperitoneum.
- Protocols: Improved documentation of vital signs while in radiology.

Preventability: Definite.

___

2) Head injury with respiratory distress

Case summary: 20-year-old female pedestrian. She arrived with BP 120/80, pulse 110, respiratory rate 14, and GCS 8. Physical exam revealed contusions on her head, but no other injuries noted. IV was started, nasal prong O_2 administered, and request for CT submitted. CT done about 2 hours later showed mild cerebral oedema. Admission to hospital was arranged. About 1 hour later (while waiting to be taken to her room), she was noted to be gurgling and to have minimal respiratory effort. Pulse oximetry revealed SaO_2 of 50%. Airway was suctioned and patient ambu-bagged. Attempts made by doctors in ED for intubation. Repeated attempts unsuccessful. During this time, SaO_2 remained persistently low. Anaesthesiologist called: difficult intubation but eventually successful. SaO_2 satisfactory after intubation. However, GCS had declined to 5. Repeat CT showed increased cerebral oedema. She was admitted to the ICU. Her neurological status continued to decline. She became unstable and expired within 24 hours. Autopsy revealed a cerebral herniation.

Discussion: The patient died from a moderate head injury, which was severely exacerbated by prolonged hypoxia. She should have been intubated early during her time in the ED. She should have had better monitoring of her vital signs, respiratory status, and oxygenation. Training for the staff in the ED, especially regarding airway management and intubation, should be improved. Deficiencies: airway management, documentation. Location of deficiency: ED.

Corrective actions:
- Targeted education: Improved training for airway management and early management of the severely injured for staff in ED, using CE, or in-service, courses (as described in section 5.1).
- Protocol development or enforcement: Improved documentation of vital sign monitoring in ED.
- System improvement/enhanced resources: Improved access to O2 saturation monitors.
- Targeted education to entire staff of ED and specific provider counselling

to those involved with this particular case: Emphasizing that patients with a decreased GCS < 8 need immediate airway intubation and that GCS 8-12 should be considered for immediate airway intubation.

- System improvement/policy or protocol development: Implementing a policy or protocol that patients with a decreased GCS < 8 need immediate airway intubation and that GCS 8-12 should be considered for immediate airway intubation.
- System improvement/policy or protocol development: Implementing a policy that patients with a GCS of < 12 must not be transported or leave the resuscitation area unless a secure airway has been established.
- Targeted education: Directed training on managing traumatic brain injuries, either a dedicated grand rounds session or another type of targeted education such as a journal club or similar educational session dedicated to management of traumatic brain injuries.

Preventability: Definite.

---

3) Death in ED from femoral artery laceration

Case summary: 20-year-old male. Records included ED note and autopsy record. The patient was in a motor vehicle crash. He was awake and alert based on bystander reports and then deteriorated rapidly with profuse bleeding by the time he was extricated. During transport by EMS, he went into cardiac arrest and was administered atropine and CPR. He died shortly after arrival at the hospital (10 minutes). ED note indicated that, by report, he had spent a long time in the field and had a prolonged extrication. An autopsy revealed a large laceration of his leg involving the right femoral artery. It also mentioned a contusion of the right lung, which was not further described.

Discussion: Deficiencies identified included haemorrhage control. It was felt that haemorrhage control could have been improved in the prehospital setting. However, there was not sufficient documentation to be sure of this. There was also lack of sufficient documentation in the ED.

Corrective actions:
- System improvement: The major corrective action identified was that of systems issues, especially improving prehospital care.
- Targeted education: Sponsor a course(s) for the region to strengthen formal prehospital training using options such PreHospital Trauma Life Support (PHTLS) or Basic Trauma Life Support (BTLS) or other equivalents.

- System improvement: There needed to be better documentation from the prehospital providers (no record was available). There might also be a need to improve capabilities for communication and response time (for instance, it seemed that a long time elapsed between the call and the arrival of the ambulance).
- System improvement: Improved capabilities for extrication (prolonged extrication was reported).
- Targeted education: Focused education and training session on haemorrhage control for prehospital providers, including practising application of direct pressure for significant or pulsatile bleeding or expanding haematoma. Additionally, this targeted education should discuss the appropriate indications and correct technique for tourniquet application for haemorrhaging from extremity injuries, which is not improved by direct pressure.

Preventability: Definite.

---

4) Delayed presentation of head injury after a pedestrian injury

Case summary: 20-year-old male. Pedestrian, hit by car. He was conscious after the event and just felt a little "banged up". He went home. Relatives reported that about a day later he started getting sleepy. At 48 hours after the injury, he became difficult to arouse and they brought him to the hospital. A CT revealed cerebral oedema and subarachnoid blood. In the ED, he was intubated after 6 hours. Initial treatment also included administration of diuretics. At 8 hours (2 hours later) he was taken to the ICU. This is where the first vital signs were recorded. Two days later, he was stable and sent to the ward and then to home. Two weeks later he was found in a stupor, and a CT scan found hydrocephalus. He underwent a ventriculostomy. No ICP was recorded. He was intubated in the ICU. He deteriorated and died 1 week later (1 month total after initial injury). An autopsy revealed herniation of the brain and bilateral pneumonia.

Discussion: Deficiencies included fluid resuscitation (giving diuretics probably not indicated). Delays in treatment (delay in treatment of cerebral oedema, also could have been intubated earlier), other (the big deficiency was that he should have had follow-up CT sooner), and documentation. Location of deficits in ED (could have been intubated sooner), ICU, ward and system inadequacy (insufficient follow-up).

Corrective actions:

- System improvement and targeted education: Improve training and capabilities in ED.
- System improvement: Improve capabilities for outpatient follow-up of discharged trauma patients.
- Improve documentation of vital signs in ED.
- Improve overall record-keeping.
- Targeted education: Dedicated training on managing traumatic brain injuries, either a dedicated grand rounds session or another type of targeted education such as a journal club or similar educational session dedicated to management of traumatic brain injuries.

Preventability: Definite.

---

5) Retroperitoneal haematoma and orthopaedic injuries in a motorcyclist, death on ICU

Case summary: 16-year-old male who was involved in a motorcycle crash. He was initially taken to a private hospital then transferred to a public hospital/ trauma centre. No vital signs were recorded prior to transfer. He was found to be unstable upon arrival and found to have a distended abdomen, normal chest and painful pelvis. He was evaluated by a surgeon. At this time his blood pressure was 70/30. He was intubated, taken to the OR where he had a negative laparotomy. Orthopaedics fixed two lower extremity fractures. He emerged from the operating room hypotensive and was taken to the ICU where he remained unstable until his death 24 hours after arrival at the hospital. Autopsy revealed a femur fracture, tibia fracture, right renal artery disruption and retroperitoneal haematoma.

Discussion: Deficiencies included haemorrhage (did not control haemorrhage), fluid resuscitation (shock for a long period of time in ED), delays in treatment, other (probably should have had DPL or ultrasound to evaluate abdomen before trip to OR for negative laparotomy; also orthopaedics should not have undertaken definitive repair of femur and tibia fracture in such an unstable patient), and documentation. Location of deficits in ED, OR (did not find or explore retroperitoneal haematoma; prolonged time for non-emergent orthopaedic procedures), interfacility transfer (no documentation, resuscitation should have been improved at referring hospital, and there is even a question as to whether he should have been transferred in such an unstable condition), and system inadequacy.

Corrective actions:

- System improvement: Improve transfer protocols and possibly transfer agreements (e.g. relations between referring and referral hospitals).
- Targeted education: Directed training on managing patients in shock, either a dedicated grand rounds session or another type of targeted education, such as a journal club or similar education session dedicated to the appropriate management and optimal resuscitation of haemodynamically unstable patients.
- Targeted teaching session or perhaps grand rounds on topic of evaluation of abdominal trauma.
- Targeted education: Training and review for providers on indications for use and technique of diagnostic peritoneal lavage to assess for haemoperitoneum.
- Systems improvement/enhanced resources: If an ultrasound machine is not already available, consideration of purchasing one or stationing one in the ED to allow for more rapid assessment for haemoperitoneum.
- Targeted education: Training and/or refresher course for providers in the use of the ultrasound (FAST exam) to quickly evaluate for intra-abdominal haemorrhage.
- Targeted education: Improve surgical expertise and equipment for exploration of retroperitoneal haematomas by arranging for surgeons to attend Definitive Surgical Trauma Care (DSTC) course, or other similar course, sponsored by hospital funds.
- Improve communication between services, in view of time taken to repair orthopaedic injuries in this unstable patient.

Preventability: Definite.

---

6) Elderly female with multiple medical problems and prolonged time in OR for fixation of fractures

Case summary: 75–year-old-female who fell down stairs at home. History of multiple medical problems. Sustained fractures of radius and ulna, shoulder, and hip. Also had change in mental status with amount of cerebral oedema on CT. Admitted to general surgery service. Taken by orthopaedics to OR on night of admission. Had 5 hours in OR for multiple orthopaedic procedures. Intermittently unstable in OR. High blood loss, required transfusions in OR. Postoperatively, developed pneumonia and multiple complications and expired on post-operative day 5.

Discussion: Should not have gone to OR on first night or should have had staged procedures performed, especially when it was clear that she was unstable. Orthopaedics had not let general surgery know that patient was going to OR. Possibly the extent of her instability and multiple medical problems had not been well communicated between the services.

Corrective actions:
- System policy change: Consulting services need to obtain clearance from primary service before taking patient to the OR.
- After this case discussed in M & M and in multidisciplinary trauma conference, a letter documenting the facts of case and the policy change should be sent to the orthopaedics service and anaesthesiology service.
- Targeted education: Directed training on managing patients in shock, either a dedicated grand rounds session or another type of targeted education such as a journal club or similar educational session dedicated to the appropriate management and optimal resuscitation of haemodynamically unstable patients.
- Targeted education: Addressing and stressing the need for "damage control" across different specialties such as general surgery, orthopaedics and anaesthesia. Targeted educational efforts such as grand rounds describing and reinforcing of the concept of "damage control" in severely injured patients with multiple injuries.

Preventability: Definite.

Section 2. **Potentially preventable death**

---

1) Multi-system organ failure after head and abdominal injury

Case summary: 50-year-old male. Sources of information were hospital record and autopsy. Motor vehicle crash. Approximately 45 minutes between event and arrival at ED. Arrival BP: 80/60; GCS 5. This patient was intubated in the ED upon arrival. He was administered crystalloid and blood for a systolic blood pressure that went below 60. A DPL was positive at approximately 20 minutes into his time in the ED. A CT of the head showed subarachnoid haemorrhage. He underwent a laparotomy 11 hours after arrival in the ED. This revealed 300 ccs of blood. He underwent a splenectomy and placement of a chest tube. There was also note of a pelvic haematoma. In the ICU, he subsequently developed multi-system organ failure, including renal failure and ARDS. He expired on day 15. An autopsy revealed 400 ccs of serous pericardial effusion.

Discussion: Discussion of this case revealed that there was probably not sufficient attention to detail as regards his abdominal work-up and his resuscitation for hypotension. Airway issues were promptly and appropriately addressed by intubation in the ED. There seemed to be an exclusive focus on his head injury initially. Deficiencies include haemorrhage control, fluid administration (probably), delays in treatment (delay in getting to operating room and bleeding control), and other (unrecognized pericardial effusion). Part of the delay in bleeding control may have been to go to the X-ray department for X-rays. Location of deficits included prehospital (possibly a little better) and ED (main issue).

Corrective actions:
- Systems improvement/enhanced resources: Improved staffing for ED, especially at peak times.
- Targeted education: Improved training for ED staff (doctors and nurses).
- Targeted education: Increased use of continuing education (CE), or in-service, courses for trauma care (as described in section 5.1), for ED staff (doctors and nurses). Such courses were available but not fully utilized.
- Targeted education: Directed training on managing patients in shock, either a dedicated grand rounds session or another type of targeted education such as a journal club or similar educational session dedicated to the appropriate management and optimal resuscitation of haemodynamically unstable patients.

Preventability: Potentially preventable.

---

2) Femur and pelvic fractures and facial lacerations

Case summary: 68-year-old male. Sources of information were medical records and autopsy. MVC. Arrived with respiratory distress and was intubated in the ED. X-rays revealed a pelvic fracture. He also had an open fracture of the femur. He went to the operating room for a plastic surgery repair of facial lacerations. There was no mention of repeat vital signs in the ED after his first BP recording of 90/40. About 24 hours later, he underwent a CT scan of the abdomen, which was normal. His blood pressure at the time was fluctuating. Haemoglobin 8. He also had increasing oxygen requirements. He died on day 6. Autopsy revealed facial lacerations, femur fracture, pelvic fracture and hydrothorax.

Discussion: Deficiencies in the patient's care included fluid resuscitation (possibly not sufficient, but not enough documentation), delays in treatment (no fracture fixation), and other (no leader in resuscitation) and documentation (not enough record of vital signs). The location of all deficits was in the ED. There seemed to be an inappropriate level of attention to the facial injury, rather than to the femur and pelvic fractures and physiological status.

Corrective actions:
- Systems improvement/enhanced resources: Improved staffing for ED, especially at peak times.
- Targeted education: Improved training for ED staff (doctors and nurses).
- Targeted education: Increased use of continuing education (CE), or in-service, courses for trauma care (as described in section 5.1), which were available but not fully utilized.
- Improved use of the concept of the "trauma team" with designated leader.
- Improved record-keeping.
- Targeted education: Directed training on managing patients in shock, either a dedicated grand rounds session or another type of targeted education such as a journal club or similar educational session dedicated to the appropriate management and optimal resuscitation of haemodynamically unstable patients.

Preventability: Potentially preventable.

---

3) Death in ED from multiple injuries

Case summary: 60-year-old male after MVC. In the ED, he was noted to have decreased blood pressure. He had a positive DPL. During his evaluation, he had a cardiac arrest and underwent CPR. He underwent thoracotomy and died in the ED. There was considerable confusion in the notes as to the times of these events. It is probable that he had decreased blood pressure for approximately 30 minutes before any action was taken. Autopsy revealed right sided rib fractures, a moderate sized right haemothorax, and liver lacerations with no mention of amount of blood.

Discussion: Deficiencies identified included haemorrhage control, fluid resuscitation, delays in treatment (ABCs not followed in face of unstable vital signs), and documentation. Location of all deficits in ED.

Corrective actions:
- Systems improvement/enhanced resources: Improved staffing for ED, especially at peak times.
- Targeted education: Improved training for ED staff (doctors and nurses).
- Targeted education: Increased use of continuing education (CE), or in-service, courses for trauma care (as described in section 5.1), which were available but not fully utilized.
- Improved use of the concept of the "trauma team" with designated leader.
- Improved record-keeping.
- Targeted education: Directed training on managing patients in shock, either a dedicated grand rounds session or another type of targeted education such as a journal club or similar educational session dedicated to the appropriate management and optimal resuscitation of haemodynamically unstable patients.

Preventability: Potentially preventable.

---

4) Death in ICU after respiratory acidosis following drainage of subdural haematoma

Case summary: 50-year-old male injured in fall from height at a construction site. At the scene he was having seizures. He was haemodynamically unstable en route but no vital signs were recorded by the paramedics. His vital signs improved from a systolic blood pressure of 80 to 120 after fluid administration in the ED. His GCS was 7. He was intubated after about 30 minutes in the ED, after having had a respiratory arrest with seizures. CT scan revealed a subdural haematoma. He was given furosemide and mannitol and was taken to OR for a craniotomy. The subdural haematoma was drained and he was taken to the ICU and died 4 hours later. He was, at the time, noted to be severely hypercarbic (PCO_2 of 75; pH 7.15). He was declared brain dead at 02:00 (6 hours after arrival). Autopsy revealed left femur and tibia fracture. Head injury included a temporal and skull-base fractures.

Discussion: Deficiencies included fluid resuscitation (diuretics not indicated in a hypotensive patient), delays in work-up (no work-up for hypotension), airway management (not intubated for 30 minutes after arrival to ED), and inadequate breathing management in light of severe respiratory acidosis at completion of OR. Location of deficits in ED plus system inadequacy (lack of leadership role in resuscitation).

Corrective actions:

- Targeted education: Improve airway management and resuscitation in ED.
- Policy: Need for improved leadership role in resuscitation.
- Improve respiratory management in OR (no ABGs obtained during the procedure), and possibly ICU.
- Targeted education: Directed training on managing traumatic brain injuries, either a dedicated grand rounds session or another type of targeted education such as a journal club or similar educational session dedicated to management of traumatic brain injuries (e.g. emphasizing basic points such as prevention of secondary brain injury, avoidance of diuretics for patients who are hypotensive).
- System improvement/policy or protocol development: Implementing a policy or protocol that patients with a decreased GCS $\leq$ 8 need immediate airway intubation and that GCS 8-12 should be considered for immediate airway intubation.
- System improvement/policy or protocol development: Implementing a policy that patient's with a GCS of $\leq$ 12 must not be transported or leave the resuscitation area unless a secure airway has been established.
- Targeted education: Directed training on managing patients in shock, either a dedicated grand rounds session or another type of targeted education such as a journal club or similar educational session dedicated to the appropriate management and optimal resuscitation of haemodynamically unstable patients.

Preventability: Potentially preventable.

---

5) Elderly man with bilateral traumatic above-knee amputations

Case summary: 75-year-old male. MVC. In the prehospital scene he was found to be in cardiac arrest and underwent CPR including defibrillation and bag valve mass respirations. He was intubated in the ED. He was noted to have bilateral above-the-knee amputations. He died approximately 15 minutes after ED arrival. Autopsy revealed no other injuries.

Discussion: Deficiencies identified included: Haemorrhage (no external haemorrhage control mentioned despite otherwise good documentation) and fluid resuscitation (possibly could have started IV and administered resuscitation but no mention of such). Location of deficits: prehospital and system inadequacies (possibly improved medical control of prehospital care).

Corrective actions:
- Systems improvement/enhanced resources: Improved capabilities for communication between field and hospital.
- Improved prehospital triage.
- Targeted education: Focused education and training session on haemorrhage control for prehospital providers, including practicing application of direct pressure for signs of significant or pulsatile bleeding or expanding haematoma. Additionally, this targeted education should discuss the appropriate indications and correct technique for tourniquet application for haemorrhaging from extremity injuries, which is not improved by direct pressure.

Preventability: Potentially preventable.

---

6) PE after chest injury

Case summary: 45-year-old male with blunt chest trauma from a motorcycle crash. Sources of information: medical record and autopsy. He had tachypnea requiring intubation in ED. Work-up revealed multiple right rib fractures and a pneumothorax, treated with a chest tube. He was admitted to the ICU for mechanical ventilation. He required 4 days on a ventilator and then was weaned off. He was in stable condition and was ready to go to the ward on face mask oxygen. He had no other injuries detected. He was on SQ heparin for DVT prophylaxis. His transfer orders from the ICU to the ward did not renew the heparin. He spent an additional day on the ICU awaiting a bed on the regular ward. The day following transfer to the regular ward, lack of DVT prophylaxis was noted. SQ heparin was restarted. About 1 day later the patient became hypotensive and short of breath. He was re-intubated and transferred back to the ICU. While a diagnostic work-up was underway, he died. Autopsy revealed a large pulmonary embolus.

Discussion: The patient went for 2 days with no DVT prophylaxis while still being bed-ridden. This was due to an omission in the orders during transfer from the ICU to the ward. As he had been receiving the prophylaxis for all of his hospital stay prior to this omission, it is not certain whether 2 additional days of SQ heparin might have changed the outcome.

Corrective actions:
- Targeted education: During the M & M meeting, the importance of DVT prophylaxis can be emphasized.

- Targeted education: Additional directed training, either a dedicated grand rounds session or another type of targeted education such as a journal club or similar educational session dedicated to DVT prophylaxis to reach a wider audience.
- Systems improvement: Discussed implementing an electronic medical record system that would automatically list the patient's existing medications that should be continued after transfer or discharge, thus minimizing the chance for error during the writing of new orders.

Preventability: Potentially preventable.

Section 3. **Death not preventable, but care could be improved**

---

1) Treatment in rural health centre before transfer for head injury

Case summary: 50-year-old male. Pedestrian injury. He was taken by bystanders to a rural health centre where he was intubated and then transferred by ambulance to the ED at the main hospital. On arrival he was noted to have a GCS of 3. He was seen by neurosurgery, who took him to the operating room to evacuate a subdural haematoma approximately 6 hours after arrival. In the ICU, he was noted to have decreased blood pressure. This intermittently fluctuated. He was also noted to have a serum sodium of 152. He died on day 2. An autopsy revealed a subdural haematoma.

Discussion: In the discussion, the neurosurgeon in the group felt that he might have been brain dead on arrival as there was mention of fixed and dilated pupils. Deficiencies in care included fluid resuscitation (no treatment of hypernatraemia; decreased blood pressure on ICU without labs being checked), care of head injury (delay of 6 hours between arrival and time of neurosurgery; possibly retained or recurrent subdural haematoma), and documentation (need for more description from autopsy). Location of deficits included prehospital care (documentation) and ICU.

Corrective actions:
- Systems improvement/enhanced resources: Strengthen ICU care, possibly through training or increased staffing.

- Counselling of the involved provider: The resident who had been on duty when the serum sodium went to 152 (without corrective action being instituted) to be informed that the review had found that this aspect of management should have been better.
- Targeted education: Directed training on managing traumatic brain injuries, either a dedicated grand rounds session or another type of targeted education such as a journal club or similar educational session dedicated to management of traumatic brain injuries.

Preventability: Not preventable, but care could be improved.

2) Extensive liver laceration

Case summary: 25-year-old female. MVC. She was hypotensive at the scene. Upon arrival to the ED she was hypotensive and had a grossly positive DPL. She was taken directly to the operating room. Laparotomy revealed a grade 5 liver laceration with 3 litre haemoperitoneum. She had a cardiac arrest in the operating room. A total of 4 units of blood had been given in the OR by the time of death. Autopsy also revealed a left haemothorax (500 ccs), for which no chest tube had been placed.

Discussion: Discussion of this case revealed no time to OR was documented in the records. Likewise, amount of fluid resuscitation and prehospital times were not documented. Deficiencies included haemorrhage (question of better control by hepatic packing instead of hepatic repair attempt). Other deficiencies included fluid resuscitation (4 units of blood not quite sufficient for grade 5 liver laceration), and lack of adequate documentation. Also, no chest tube was placed despite the haemothorax. In general, life-saving X-rays (chest and pelvis) should be performed within minutes of arrival. Location of deficit included ED and OR (mainly).

Corrective actions:
- Targeted education: Care providers, doctors and nursing staff instructed on importance of keeping track of fluid resuscitation, especially in ED.
- Targeted education: Directed training on managing patients in shock, either a dedicated grand rounds session or another type of targeted education such as a journal club or similar educational session dedicated to the appropriate management and optimal resuscitation of haemodynamically unstable patients.

- Targeted education: Grand rounds or interactive discussion session on abdominal trauma (management of complex liver injuries and use of damage-control trauma surgery).
- Develop institutional protocol on indications for chest tube placement in patients with evidence of pneumothorax or haemothorax.

Preventability: Not preventable, but care could have been better (chest tube placed, different technique for repair of liver).

---

3) Liver laceration and colon injury in a motorcyclist; death in OR

Case summary: 30-year-old male who was a motorcyclist. There were no prehospital data. He arrived with a GCS of 3, with severe hypotension (BP60/0). He was resuscitated in the ED. DPL was grossly positive. He was taken quickly to the OR for a laparotomy which revealed a grade 3 liver laceration (1500 ccs blood), and a retroperitoneal haematoma. He died approximately half an hour after being in the operating room and a total of 1.5 hours after arrival at the hospital. Operative notes indicate that at the time of his death the surgeons were undertaking a repair of his colon laceration. Autopsy revealed bilateral rib fracture, lung contusion and laceration, 500 ccs haemopneumothorax, cardiac contusion, colon laceration, retroperitoneal haematoma (no cause mentioned).

Discussion: Deficiencies included haemorrhage (delayed control of haemorrhage, possibly attention should have been directed first towards liver and retroperitoneal haematoma rather than colon laceration), chest (need for chest tube), fluid resuscitation (probably low volume compared to need, but difficult to know from records), and documentation. Location of deficits: ED and OR.

Corrective actions:
- Improve documentation of prehospital vital signs.
- Improve overall record-keeping.
- Targeted education: Directed training on managing patients in shock, either a dedicated grand rounds session or another type of targeted education such as a journal club or similar educational session dedicated to the appropriate management and optimal resuscitation of haemodynamically unstable patients.
- Targeted education: Grand rounds or interactive discussion session with topic being abdominal trauma (management of complex liver injuries and use of damage-control trauma surgery).

- Develop institutional protocol for indications for chest tube placement in patients with evidence of pneumothorax or haemothorax.

Preventability: Not preventable, but care could be improved.

---

4) Prolonged extrication, mesenteric avulsion, and cardiac arrest

Case summary: 60-year-old male, MVC. There was no prehospital record for review. However, the ED notes reported that he had been trapped in the vehicle and had undergone a prolonged extrication. He was agitated and pale on arrival. He went into asystole in the ED and was intubated with CPR. He recovered a cardiac rhythm and a BP of 60/0. He went to the operating room 30 minutes after arrival where a 3-liter haemoperitoneum was found. There was mesenteric avulsion. He was transfused 10 liters of blood. He died in the OR 6 hours after arrival. Autopsy revealed a retroperitoneal haematoma and root of mesentery tear.

Discussion: Deficiencies included haemorrhage (could a damage control laparotomy have been done instead?), delays in treatment (question of more prompt arrival at OR, although 30 minutes is already fairly short), documentation, and systems issues (delays in obtaining prehospital care, possible need for improvement of capabilities for extrication). Also note that the only records for this case were the ED notes and the autopsy. There was no operating room note in the records. Location of deficits prehospital, and OR.

Corrective actions:
- Improve prehospital capabilities, especially as regards extrication.
- Improve documentation of prehospital vital signs.
- Improve overall documentation.
- Counselling for involved providers: Discuss the need for more use of damage-control laparotomy for severely unstable trauma patients.
- Targeted education: Directed training on managing patients in shock and on damage control techniques, either a dedicated grand rounds session or another type of targeted education such as a journal club or similar educational session dedicated to the appropriate management and optimal resuscitation of haemodynamically unstable patients.
- Targeted education: Improve surgical expertise for management of mesenteric injuries and of retroperitoneal haematomas by arranging for surgeons to attend Definitive Surgical Trauma Care (DSTC) course, or other similar course, sponsored by hospital funds.

Preventability: Not preventable, but care could be improved.

5) Elderly male pedestrian in rural area

Case summary: 80-year-old male. He was a pedestrian injured in a rural area. The event appeared to occur at 20:00 (8 PM). He arrived at the ED at 23:00 (11 PM). There were no prehospital data. It was not even noted whether he arrived by car or by ambulance. He was noted to have rib fractures and a deep laceration of the leg, which was treated with a pressure dressing. He was intubated and given IV fluids. A half-hour after arrival, he was taken to the operating room where he was noted to have a weak pulse and no detectable blood pressure. Exploratory laparotomy revealed a grade 1 liver laceration with 300 ccs of blood. There was an open femur fracture and a popliteal vessel injury. He died in the OR 4 hours after arrival. Autopsy revealed a small subdural haematoma and right rib fractures with a pneumothorax. It should also be noted there was no mention of a chest X-ray in the emergency room.

Discussion: Deficiencies included chest (no chest tube), delays in treatment (delay in transport to hospital), and documentation. Location of deficits: prehospital (very prolonged prehospital time), ED (no chest X-ray), no treatment for pneumothorax and system inadequacy (prehospital care and time).

Corrective actions:
- Improve prehospital documentation.
- Improve ED documentation.
- Targeted education: Increased use of continuing education (CE), or in-service, courses for trauma care (as described in section 5.1), which were available but not fully utilized.
- Develop institutional protocol on indications for chest tube placement in patients with evidence of pneumothorax or haemothorax.
- Targeted education: Directed training on managing patients in shock and on damage control techniques, either a dedicated grand rounds session or another type of targeted education such as a journal club or similar educational session dedicated to the appropriate management and optimal resuscitation of haemodynamically unstable patients.

Preventability: Not preventable, but care could be improved.

Section 4. **Death not preventable**

1) Death in OR with liver and spleen injuries

Case summary: 20-year-old male after MVC. Intubated in the ED. BP 80/40 on arrival. Open forearm fracture noted. DPL positive and taken to operating room. Severe splenic injury and grade 4 hepatic injuries noted. Total blood loss 4000 ccs. Splenectomy undertaken. The patient died in the OR. He had been taken to the OR about 1 hour after arrival. Diagnostic burr holes were performed in the operating room as there had not been time for a CT scan given his hypotension and positive DPL. No mention was made in the ED records of amount of fluid given. In the OR he had 6 litres of crystalloid and 4 units of blood.

Discussion: In theory, all of the injuries should have been survivable with proper treatment. There were some items of care that could have been improved to some extent. For example, he might have been taken to the OR in less than 1 hour. Fluid resuscitation in the ED could have been better documented (none was documented). In the operating room, decision-making might have been better in the form of a damage-control laparotomy. However, these mostly seemed to be small improvements that would have been unlikely to have resulted in his survival.

Corrective actions: None needed.

Preventability: Not preventable.

2) GSW to abdomen with cardiac arrest

Case summary: 25-year-old male with gunshot wound to abdomen. Source of information: medical record. Initially with pulse and BP then arrested in ED. Left thoracotomy performed in ED – no tamponade or cardiac or pulmonary injury. Aorta cross-clamped with restoration of blood pressure. Taken emergently to OR for laparotomy. Found to have a large liver laceration and small and large bowel injuries. He underwent a damage control laparotomy during which his liver was packed and the small and large bowel lacerations oversewn. He was taken to ICU coagulopathic and hypothermic. Continued to bleed even after coagulopathy corrected. Became progressively more hypotensive and died.

Discussion: Severe injury, treatment appropriate.

Corrective actions: None needed.

Preventability: Not preventable.

---

3) PE after multiple orthopaedic injuries

Case summary: 40-year-old female, MVC. Source of information: medical record and autopsy. Had multiple orthopaedic injuries. Stable on arrival and in ED. No respiratory distress. Taken to OR for ORIF of femur fracture and placement of external fixator on day of injury. Postoperative orders were written for SQ heparin and sequential compression devices for DVT prophylaxis. On second postoperative day, patient became progressively more short of breath with intermittent hypotension. Suspicion of PE. Patient was given bolus of heparin. Cardiac arrest on way to ventilation-perfusion scan. CPR, without success. Patient expired. Autopsy revealed a saddle-type pulmonary embolus.

Discussion: Severe complication, treatment appropriate.

Corrective action: None needed.

Preventability: Not preventable.

---

4) Blunt cardiac injury and multiple abdominal injuries

Case summary: 70-year-old female, pedestrian injury. Source of information: medical record. Hypotensive in the ED with grossly positive DPL and pelvic fracture. Taken to the OR where severe hepatic injuries were packed. Cardiac arrest in OR, left thoracotomy performed with cardiac massage. Cardiac rhythm returned. Taken to ICU where multiple pressors required for cardiogenic shock, thought to be due to underlying cardiac disease or to blunt cardiac injury. Vital signs stabilized, pressors decreased. On second hospital data, it was noted that patient was not moving (had come into ED moving, though with decreased consciousness and had an initially normal head CT). Repeat CT showed large bilateral strokes, probably secondary to prolonged hypotension. No return of neurological function. Developed multi-system organ system failure and died.

Discussion: Severe injury, treatment appropriate.

Corrective actions: None needed.

Preventability: Not preventable.

Section 5. Non-fatal cases, but problems identified that required corrective actions

1) Infected impalement wound

Case summary: 20-year-old male, fall at construction site. Laceration to left thigh from impalement on iron bar. No fracture. Neurovascular status intact distally. Taken to OR for debridement and closure by residents at night. Two days later developed fever, tachycardia, erythema around wound. Sutures DC'd; pus drained, but muscles seemed dark. Taken back to OR for further debridement. Myonecrosis identified, along with retained debris, including pieces of cloth. Extensive debridement performed. Patient septic, prolonged course with multiple repeat operations, but eventually recovered.

Discussion: Preventable complication. Patient should have had more extensive debridement in OR on first occasion. Probably also should have had wound left open rather than closed. Hence, error in technique. Also, systems issue – need for more attending (senior) presence for major debridements in OR.

Corrective actions:
- Targeted education: During M & M conference, residents instructed on need for complete debridement of dirty wounds and avoidance of primary closure in these circumstances.
- System and policy change: Attendings (specialists, consultants, faculty) instructed on need to be present for and directly participate in such cases.

Preventability: Potentially preventable.

2) Retained haemothorax

Case summary: 50-year-old male, fall from height. Multiple left rib fractures. Spent one week in hospital and was discharged. Small pleural effusion evident at time of admission. This enlarged on subsequent days. Patient was doing well at time of clinic visit. Slightly decreased breath sounds at left base noted, but no chest X-ray obtained. Patient returned 1 month later with increased shortness of breath. CXR showed much larger pleural effusion. Admitted for chest tube placement, minimal amount of serosanguinous fluid obtained. Patient eventually required decortication for retained haemothorax and trapped lung. Had 2-week hospitalization, but eventually recovered.

Discussion: Pleural effusion was evident at initial hospitalization and should have been drained as it was likely to represent haemothorax. Another missed opportunity for draining this before it became fibrosed was at his 1-week follow-up in clinic.

Corrective actions:
- Targeted education: Residents instructed on consequences of retained haemothorax and need for more prompt drainage of traumatic pleural effusions.
- Develop institutional protocol for indications for chest tube placement in patients with evidence of pneumothorax or haemothorax.

Preventability: Potentially preventable.